LECTURE NOTES
Neurology

IVAN T. DRAPER
MB, ChB, FRCPE
*Neurologist, Institute of
Neurological Sciences and
Western Infirmary,
Glasgow*

FIFTH EDITION

BLACKWELL
SCIENTIFIC PUBLICATIONS
OXFORD LONDON EDINBURGH
BOSTON MELBOURNE

To MMD

© 1965, 1968, 1970, 1974, 1980 by
Blackwell Scientific Publications
Editorial offices:
Osney Mead, Oxford, OX2 0EL
8 John Street, London, WC1N 2ES
9 Forrest Road, Edinburgh, EH1 2QH
52 Beacon Street, Boston,
   Massachusetts 02108, USA
214 Berkeley Street, Carlton
   Victoria 3053, Australia

All rights reserved. No part of this
publication may be reproduced, stored
in a retrieval system, or transmitted,
in any form or by any means,
electronic, mechanical, photocopying,
recording or otherwise
without the prior permission of
the copyright owner

First published 1965
Second edition 1968
Third edition 1970
Fourth edition 1974
Reprinted 1976, 1978
Fifth edition 1980

Set printed and bound in Great Britain
by Billing and Sons Limited,
Guildford, London, Oxford, Worcester

DISTRIBUTORS

USA
   Blackwell Mosby Book Distributors
   11830 Westline Industrial Drive
   St Louis, Missouri 63141

Canada
   Blackwell Mosby Book Distributors
   120 Melford Drive, Scarborough
     Ontario, M1B 2X4

Australia
   Blackwell Scientific Book
   Distributors
   214 Berkeley Street, Carlton
   Victoria 3053

British Library
Cataloguing in Publication Data

Draper, Ivan Thomas
   Lecture notes on neurology. – 5th ed.
   1. Nervous system – Diseases
   I. Title
   616.8   RC346   80-40632

ISBN 0-632-00572-6

Contents

	PAGE
Preface	vii

Part I: The Structure and Function of the Nervous System

1 The Motor System — 3
   The Corticospinal Pathway. Co-ordinated Movement. Muscle Tone
2 Sensation — 19
3 The Autonomic Nervous System — 23
4 Cranial Nerves — 29
5 Functional Topography of the Brain — 44
6 Cerebral Circulation — 50
7 Spinal Cord — 52
8 Cerebrospinal Fluid — 55
9 Consciousness — 58
10 Higher Functions: Speech and Memory — 60

Part II: The History and Examination — 63

Part III: Diseases of the Nervous System

11 Epilepsy — 83
12 Cerebral Palsy — 95
13 Head Injury — 97
14 Intracranial Tumour — 101

		PAGE
15	Infections of the Nervous System	108
	Brain Abscess. Bacterial Meningitis. Neurosyphilis. Virus Infections.	
16	Cerebrovascular Disease	122
17	Organic Dementia	132
18	Diseases of the Basal Ganglia	136
19	Headache	142
20	Facial Pain	146
21	Facial Palsy	149
22	Labyrinthine Vertigo	151
23	The Differential Diagnosis of Disease of the Spinal Cord	152
24	Compression of the Spinal Cord	156
	Spinal Cord Tumour. Cervical Spondylosis.	
25	Subacute Combined Degeneration of the Cord	162
26	Motor Neuron Disease	165
27	Syringomyelia	169
28	The Demyelinating Diseases	172
29	The Hereditary Ataxias	179
30	The Care of the Paraplegic Patient	179
31	Prolapsed Intervertebral Disc	181
32	The Neuropathies	183
33	Myasthenia Gravis	193
34	Diseases of the Muscle	196
35	The Non-Metastatic Complications of Carcinoma	203
	Suggestions for Further Reading	205
	Index	206

Preface

Clinical neurology is founded upon the analysis of an accurate history and examination, interpreted in the light of a knowledge of anatomy and of the common neurological illnesses. These notes are intended to provide a basis for this exercise. They were designed for use in conjunction with a formal course of instruction and as a means of rapid revision. This format imposes limitations on the amount of detail which can be provided and it makes no allowance for controversial opinions. My approach to neurology owes a great deal to my own teachers, especially to Professor J.A. Simpson and the late Dr J.B. Stanton, and to my colleagues at the Institute and elsewhere.

I.T.D.

Part I
The Structure and Function of the Nervous System

Chapter 1
The Motor System: Organization and Function

The complexity of human behaviour, the range of man's imagination, the accuracy of his perception, his speech and the precision and power of his movements are products of a normally functioning nervous system. The basic unit of the nervous system is the nerve cell or neuron of which there are 10–50,000,000 000. The neuron is a relatively simple structure whose response is limited to the generation of a standard impulse. The variety and adaptability of neural function is achieved by the almost limitless number of connections which exist between the neurons. Each neuron has several fibrous projections, one of which, the axon transmits the impulse generated in the nerve cell body. There are several branching dendrites from which stubby spines project. These form the receptor surfaces for the synapses between one neuron and the next. The spines can accumulate energy from a number of subthreshold stimuli from one axon or from different axons. Eventually the spine discharges and an impulse is transmitted to the cell body. This mechanism of cumulative responses adds spatial and temporal dimensions to neuronal activity. Chains and networks of neurons are activated for various receptor (sensory) and effector (motor) functions.

The execution of precise rapid movement depends on the integrated activity of the whole nervous system, both sensory and motor. It is the custom to divide the motor system into pyramidal and extrapyramidal parts, but it is wrong to equate this division with voluntary and involuntary mechanisms. Of the pyramidal tract fibres, only a quarter originate in the motor cortex, while the rest come from the parietal lobe and the basal–reticular complex. On the other hand, the extrapyramidal system is responsible for a great proportion of voluntary and semi-voluntary movement, particularly the learned and habitual movements, and those associated with posture. Thus the fibres arising from the giant cells of the *motor cortex* are responsible for consciously willed activity, such as the control of fine, unfamiliar hand movements. For such action to be effective it must be superimposed on the pre-existing postural patterns established by the activity of the basal–reticular system.

The somatic structures are represented over the cortical motor strip, which lies anterior to the central sulcus of the brain (Fig. 1). Electrical stimulation of this area causes movement in the equivalent contralateral part of the body.

The corticospinal tract, comprising fibres from the motor cortex and the parietal lobe, passes down through the internal capsule to the brain-stem. Here it is joined by fibres from the basal ganglia and reticular formation. In the medulla they are grouped into well-defined bundles called the pyramids, and here the major decussation (crossing) occurs. In the spinal cord the crossed pyramidal tracts lie lateral to the central grey matter. The individual fibres finally synapse with the anterior horn cells of the cord, either directly or through one or more interneurons.

The *extrapyramidal system* is less clearly defined. Fibres from the motor cortex synapse with the cells of the basal ganglia, thalamus and reticular formation. Apart from the contribution of

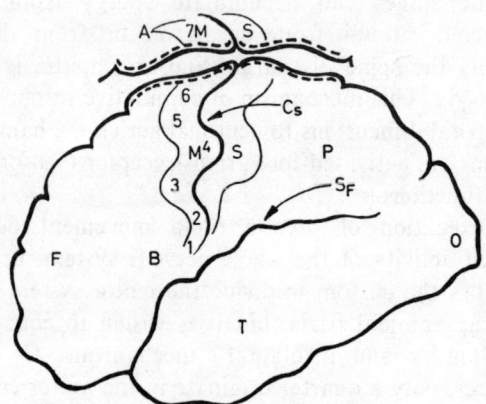

Fig. 1. Lateral view of the left cerebral hemisphere, with the adjacent part of the medial surface shown inset.

A. Accessory motor area. B. Broca's area. Cs. Central sulcus. F. Frontal lobe. M. Motor cortex. O. Occipital lobe. P. Parietal lobe. S. Sensory cortex. Sf. Sylvian fissure. T. Temporal lobe.

Representation of the body over the motor cortex.

1. Mouth. 2. Face. 3. Thumb. 4. Hand. 5. Arm. 6. Trunk. 7. Leg.

fibres to the pyramidal tracts, the majority travel to the cord by the reticulospinal and rubrospinal pathways. The final synapse is with the anterior horn cells, particularly those of the gamma system. Due to the large number of synapses the extrapyramidal system conducts impulses slowly, but by the same token, complex patterns of nerve and muscle activity can be initiated.

Functionally, it is convenient to think of the cerebral cortex influencing and modifying the action of the basal ganglia, which in turn modify the centres of the brain-stem, in turn modifying the cord reflexes. At every level there is a feedback of 'information' to the higher centres (Fig. 2). The cerebellum is a monitor in this feedback network. Disease, at any level in the motor system, releases the centres below from the influence of those above. In determining the level or site of a lesion, the concepts of an upper motor neuron and a lower motor neuron are used.

The upper motor neuron should be thought of as all the descending fibres, both corticospinal and reticulospinal, which

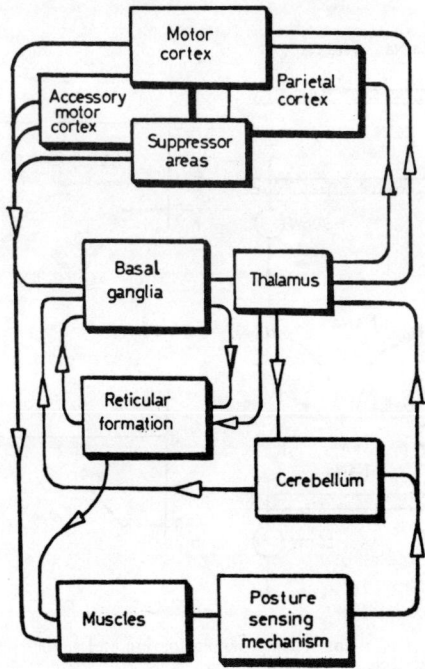

Fig. 2. Block diagram of the motor control system with feedback pathways.

influence the anterior horn cells. The lower motor neuron is the final common path in the motor system, the anterior horn cell of the cord and its axon extending out in the peripheral nerve.

The normal function of the *peripheral nerve* is dependent upon the 'health' of its parent cell body and the integrity of the axon and its myelin sheath. Disordered metabolism in the cell is thus manifest by functional failure at the periphery. Nerve conduction studies provide a method for the in-vivo study of motor nerve function. Each anterior horn cell innervates several muscle fibres. The cell, the axon, its branches and the muscle fibres are termed a motor unit.

The *neuromuscular junction* is bridged by the release of acetylcholine. The arrival of a nerve impulse causes the discharge of minute quantities of acetylcholine from vesicles near the nerve ending. These combine briefly with the receptor protein of the motor end plate—a specialized part of the muscle membrane.

At rest, the inside of the muscle cell carries a negative charge (—90 mV) with respect to the surrounding tissue fluid (Fig. 3a).

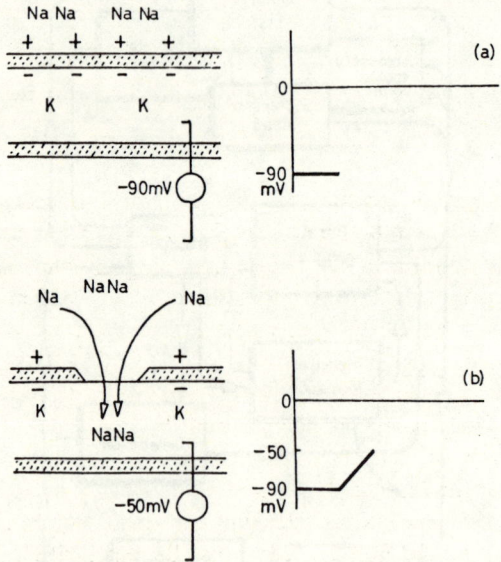

Fig. 3 The sequences of events during depolarization and repolarization.
Fig. 3a. The resting, polarized cell.
Fig. 3b. Acetylcholine causes a local reduction in the membrane potential. Sodium ions begin to flow into the cell.

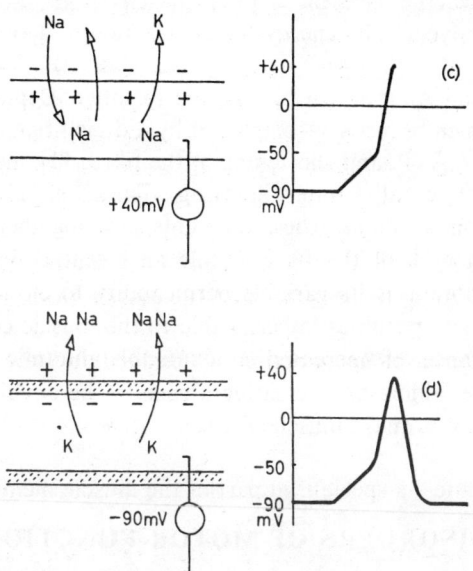

Fig. 3. The sequences of events during depolarization and repolarization.
Fig. 3c. Accumulation of positively charged ions within the cell makes the interior of the fibre locally positive. 'Depolarization'.
Fig. 3d. Sodium ions are expelled from the cell by an active pump mechanism. Repolarization.

In other words, it is polarized. The cellular fluid contains a high concentration of potassium (157 mEq l^{-1}) and a low concentration of sodium (14 mEq l^{-1}). The arrival of acetylcholine induces a reduction in the membrane potential to about -50 mV (Fig. 3b). This increases the permeability of the membrane to the positively charged sodium ions which flow into the cell. The inside of the cell now carries a positive charge ($+40$ mV). It is depolarized (Fig. 3c). Thus, partial depolarization by acetylcholine at the end plate induces a self-generating wave of depolarization which spreads over the muscle membrane.

During this time the muscle fibre contracts. Before the fibre can respond again, the muscle cells must be repolarized. This occurs when the acetylcholine is broken down by an enzyme cholinesterase which is normally present at the neuromuscular junctiton. The electrolyte constituents of the cell are returned to their resting concentrations by an active pump mechanism (Fig. 3d).

The contractile element of the *muscle fibre* is a combined protein actomycin. The energy for contraction is derived from the breakdown of adenosine triphosphate (ATP). At rest, the actomycin and ATP are firmly bonded together. Depolarization of the muscle membrane is accompanied by a dissolution of this bond, breakdown of ATP, and shortening of the fibre. The muscle fibre is composed of parallel interdigitating filaments. The effect of depolarization is to make these filaments slide together, shortening the overall length of the fibre. While an essential feature of the muscle membrane is its variable permeability to electrolytes, it is for all practical purposes impermeable to the muscle cell enzymes. The appearance of increased amounts of glutamic oxaloacetic transaminase, aldolase, or creatine kinase in the circulating blood, is indicative of primary muscle disease.

DISORDERS OF MOTOR FUNCTION

Disorders of motor function are manifested by three main groups of symptoms:
> weakness;
> incoordination and involuntary movements;
> altered tone.

Weakness

Weakness results from an interruption in the motor pathway at any level, affecting the upper or lower motor neutron, the neuromuscular junction or the muscle.

(1) Upper motor neuron lesions

An upper motor neuron lesion causes weakness of willed movements and it releases irrelevant patterns of muscular tone (spasticity). In health, this hypertonicity is inhibited by the influence of the corticoreticular fibres. The distribution of hypertonic muscles in a 'spastic' limb is not a consequence of haphazard neuronal activity. The extended legs and the flexed adducted arms represent the re-emergence of primitive supporting postures which had been modified by subsequent neuronal maturation.

The weakness is likely to affect movements rather than

individual muscles. Thus, a muscle may be weak or paralysed for the execution of one movement but retain normal power when used in a different movement, e.g. there may be paralysis of voluntary wrist extension, while the same muscles act powerfully as synergists when the patient clenches his fist. Fine, highly differentiated movements, e.g. digital manipulation, are likely to be more severely affected than coarse proximal movements. Muscle tone is increased. The tendon reflexes are brisk and clonus may be present. The plantar reflexes, if involved, are extensor. Muscle wasting occurs only after a delay and is due to disuse. There is no fasciculation.

A destructive or compressive lesion at any level in the brain or spinal cord may be responsible.

Cortical lesions cause contralateral paralysis. Due to the dispersion of the cortical representation a discrete lesion in the motor cortex will give rise to a circumscribed paresis.

Lesions in the *internal capsule* (a common site for cerebral haemorrhage) are likely to cause a complete contralateral hemiparesis as the descending fibres here are grouped closely together.

Brain-stem lesions often affect both corticospinal tracts. If sited above the mid pons they may cause a pseudobulbar palsy. This consists of a spastic weakness of the facial muscles, the muscles of mastication, the tongue and palate. The jaw jerk is increased, the tongue lies stiffly in the floor of the mouth, and there is a spastic dysarthria. Motiveless crying or laughter frequently accompanies a pseudobulbar palsy.

A lesion of the corticospinal tract below the pyramidal decussation gives rise to an ipsilateral spastic paralysis. See Brown-Séquard syndrome (p. 55).

(2) Lower motor neuron lesions

The weakness is likely to involve specific muscles or groups of muscles for all movements. Muscle tone is decreased. The tendon reflexes are depressed or lost early in the disease. The plantar reflexes, if present, are flexor. Muscle wasting occurs early and is prominent. Fasciculation may occur.

Fasciculation is the brief subcutaneous rippling movement seen over the muscle bellies. It is caused by momentary shock-like contractions of the muscle fibres comprising one motor unit.

Disease of the nerve cell body or the proximal part of the axon generates abnormal motor impulses which activate these fibres.

Fibrillation is the spontaneous contraction of single muscle fibres. It is an electromyographic diagnosis and cannot be recognized clinically.

Lower motor neuron signs are likely to be found at the site of any lesion in the brain-stem or spinal cord, combined with upper neuron signs below the level of the lesion. Lesions of the anterior horn cells, nerve roots or peripheral nerves cause isolated lower neuron lesions with a specific distribution. Nerve conduction studies and electromyography may be of assistance in locating the lesion.

Symmetrical, peripheral, lower neuron weakness is described in the section on the neuropathies. Isolated lower neuron weakness is most commonly due to local compression. Neurotropic virus infection and exposure to toxic chemicals are less frequently responsible.

(3) Neuromuscular junction

Myasthenia gravis is the only spontaneously occurring example of a disorder at this site. The outstanding feature is a rapid loss of power on sustained or repeated contraction of the muscle, which may be restored to normal by the administration of anticholinesterase drugs.

Affected muscles are hypotonic, yet the tendon reflexes are normal or brisk. Wasting is a late feature and fasciculation only occurs as a result of over-treatment.

(4) Muscle

Primary muscle disease often causes symmetrical weakness, affecting the proximal muscles more than the distal ones. Wasting occurs, but is usually less prominent than the weakness, and tendon reflexes are diminished only in proportion to the wasting. Fasciculation does not occur except in thyrotoxic myopathy (p. 201). Electromyography is usually diagnostic. Serum muscle enzymes are raised if the process is active. In the group of inherited muscle disorders (the muscular dystrophies) a family history may be obtained.

Co-ordinated movement

The performance of an unfamiliar manual task requires conscious effort. The initial attempts are slow, stiff and imprecise and fatigue rapidly. With practice these defects are reversed and the action is absorbed into the individual's programme of motor skills. Such a learning process probably involves physical changes in the neurons concerned so that the flow of impulses along a specific pathway is facilitated. Repetition enhances the facilitation.

Fully co-ordinated movements depend on:
1. The cerebral cortex for the organization and analysis of willed movements.
2. The basal ganglia for the semi-voluntary and postural patterned movements.
3. The motor system for the execution of movement.
4. The sensory system to provide constant inflow of information regarding posture, orientation and position of the limbs.
5. The cerebellum to co-ordinate the sensory input. It is then matched against the cortical pattern of required activity and the appropriate modifications are made through the extrapyramidal system (Fig. 2).

(1) Cerebral cortex

The conscious ordering of movement is sometimes called praxis. It depends on the individual's ability to retain the pattern and sequence of a required movement and to translate instructions or intentions into effect. The seat of this cortical organization is in the dominant parietal lobe, from where there are subcortical connections with the motor cortex. The control of cortically organized movements crosses to the non-dominant hemisphere via the corpus callosum.

Disorders of consciously organized patterns of movement are termed apraxias. There is no paralysis, sensory disturbance or ataxia, and the patient fully understands the nature of his task. It is as though his 'memory' for organizing the correct sequence of movements were lost. Movements are performed awkwardly and the patient is often unable to gesture or use simple mechanical instruments such as scissors. Apraxia is closely related to some forms of motor dysphasia.

(2) Basal ganglia

The basal ganglia are nuclear masses buried deeply in the white matter of the cerebral cortex. They form the anterior and lateral relations of the thalamus from which they are separated by the internal capsule (Figs 4, 4a, 4b). Afferent fibres to the basal ganglia come from the motor and supplementary motor areas of the cortex; from the parietal lobe; from the auditory and visual cortex; from the cerebellum and so indirectly from the vestibular

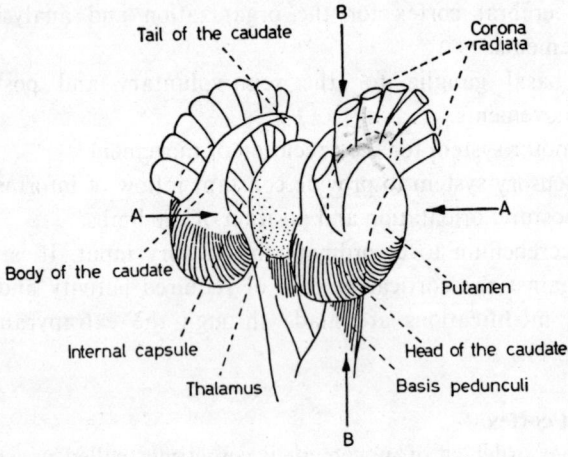

Fig. 4. The basal ganglia and adjacent structures seen obliquely from the front.

system, the postural sensing mechanism of the limbs and the neck muscles.

Both voluntary stimuli and postural reflexes modify the activity of the basal ganglia. Some influences facilitate and some are inhibitory. Facilitatory influences and the outflow from the basal ganglia are mediated by acetylcholine. The substantia nigra has an inhibitory effect which is mediated by dopamine. The major outflow from the basal ganglia is from the globus pallidus to the ventro-lateral nucleus of the thalamus and thence to the reticular formation. At every level there are feedback pathways to those above so that the output is constantly modified.

There are contributions to the pyramidal tract, but the main extrapyramidal outflow is by the reticulospinal and rubrospinal tracts. There are also connections with the interstitial nuclei, and so with the descending fibres of the medial longitudinal fasciculus (Fig. 16).

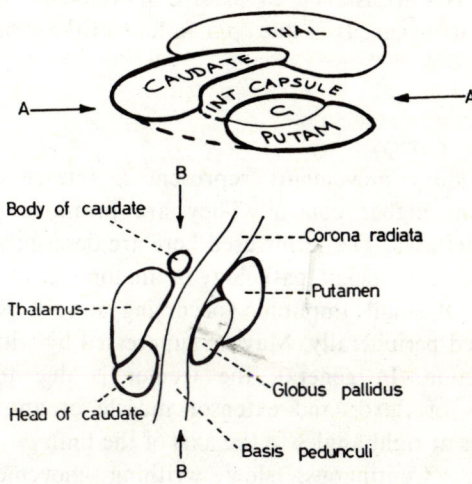

Fig. 4a. Horizontal section through the basal ganglia of the left side at A—A.
Fig. 4b. Vertical section through the basal ganglia of the left side at B—B.

The basal ganglia are largely responsible for the organization of involuntary and semi-voluntary activity upon which consciously willed movements are superimposed. Many movements which at first must be learnt with painstaking effort are eventually performed without conscious thought, and become part of the repertoire of the basal ganglia.

The basal ganglia are also responsible for supplementary movements. These include the associated movements and the control of antagonists and synergists. The associated movements supplement voluntary action largely for the maintenance of balance, e.g. swinging the arms while walking.

Disease of the basal ganglia results in two contrasting groups of symptoms. One is typified by a reduction in the supportive movements and the other by superfluous motor activity.

Reduced activity

Bradykinesia is a slowness in initiating and maintaining movements.

Loss of associated movements. The arms hang still by the patient's side, the speech is monotonous, the face is expressionless. Corrective movements are lost so that the patient tends to fall. The gait is shuffling with small steps.

Rigidity is a resistance to passive movements which persists throughout its range. It is due to a failure in the inhibition of the antagonists.

Superfluous activity
The involuntary movements represent a release of patterned activity from higher control. They are primitive postural and contactual reflexes. The terms used here are descriptive and do not refer to specific aetiology, pathology or anatomical site.

Tremor. Of small amplitude, occurring at rest. Rate 4-6 s^{-1}. Most marked peripherally. May be suppressed by will, or vigorous physical action. In general, the tremor is due to alternating contractions of flexor and extensor muscle groups, so that the movement is at right angles to the axis of the limb.

Athetosis. Continuous, slow writhing movements, chiefly affecting the distal part of the limbs. The movements are mainly rotatory, around the long axis of the affected limb. The hand often adopts a posture with the digits hyperextended, the thumb opposed, and with varying degrees of flexion at the metacarpophalangeal joints.

Hemiballismus. A violent, throwing movement. Usually restricted to one arm. The proximal musculature is primarily involved.

Chorea. Sudden, jerky movements affecting the face and arms more often than the legs. While the initial movement is very fast, the latter part is often slowed, so that a new posture will be held for a moment or two giving the impression of some purpose.

Dystonia. A rare syndrome in which distorted postures are maintained for long periods. The distortion is based upon rotation and adduction of the limbs and extension of the spine.

Myoclonus. It accompanies disease of the reticular formation or cerebellum. It is a brief, jerking movement of the limbs frequently associated with epilepsy.

(3) Disorders of motor function have already been discussed (p. 8).

(4) Sensory system

The sensory fibres in the peripheral nerves and spinal cord carry a constant flow of information about the postural disposition of the limbs and joints. An interruption of these afferent pathways necessitates dependence on the visual monitoring of position. Thus, incoordination is more apparent when the patient closes his eyes.

Peripheral nerve lesions (e.g. polyneuropathies) make it difficult for the patient to handle small objects. Lesions of the posterior root ganglia (e.g. tabes dorsalis) and posterior columns of the spinal cord (e.g. subacute combined degeneration of the cord) interfere with muscle/joint position sense. The ataxic gait is then more pronounced when the patient closes his eyes (Rombergism).

(5) The cerebellum

The cerebellum regulates the postural reflexes and muscle tone in response to varying physical activity and thus maintains the body's equilibrium. Its normal function is essential also for the performance of smoothly co-ordinated voluntary actions.

The cerebellum lies in the posterior fossa of the skull and forms the roof of the 4th ventricle. It comprises three main lobes, anterior, middle and posterior. The anterior and posterior lobes are small, mainly mid-line structures and are together known as the palaeocerebellum. The middle lobe is large and forms the greater part of the cerebellar hemispheres. There is little significant decussation within the cerebellum. The cerebellum is connected with the brain-stem by three pairs of fibre bundles, the superior, middle and inferior cerebellar peduncles.

Afferent fibres reach the cerebellum along all three pairs of cerebellar peduncles and terminate in the cerebellar cortex. The large Purkinje cells form the connection between the cortex and the cerebellar nuclei (dentate, globose, emboliform and fastigial nuclei) whence the efferent fibres are derived.

Afferent impulses from the vestibular system, the eyes and the muscle/joint receptors of the lower limbs and trunk are integrated by the palaeocerebellum. This then modifies motor activity via the basal ganglia to maintain the body's postural stability. The middle lobe of the cerebellum receives the bulk of its afferent fibres from the cerebral motor cortex via the pontine nuclei. Voluntary movements are co-ordinated so that they are performed with economy of effort and precision.

A discrete lesion in one cerebellar hemisphere gives rise to signs and symptoms which are limited to the same side of the body. The fine voluntary movements are especially affected. There is a decomposition of movements (intention tremor) and an inability to apply the appropriate force to achieve a target (overshoot). The affected limb is ataxic and the muscles are hypotonic. Nystagmus is usually prominent.

A lesion involving the mid-line cerebellar structures (palaeocerebellum) chiefly affects the maintenance of equilibrium and the postural controls associated with locomotion. There is seldom any dysfunction which can be recognized when the patient is examined in bed, but his tottering gait and broad-based stance make it apparent when he tries to stand.

Symptoms of cerebellar disease

(*a*) Voluntary movements, instead of being smooth, are irregular and broken up. The apparent seeking movements become wilder when nearing the target (intention tremor). Inappropriate force is employed and the checking mechanism is defective so that there is overshoot (dysmetria). Handwriting is typically large and irregular.

(*b*) Rapidly alternating movements are wild and irregular (dysdiadochokinesia). This is the result of imperfect modulation of the activity of agonists and antagonists.

(*c*) Speech is slurred and sometimes 'scanning'. In this form of dysarthria the syllables are separated, so that the speech is reminiscent of a child reciting poetry.

(*d*) Cerebellar nystagmus is coarse and jerky. The amplitude is greatest when the patient looks towards the side of the lesion.

(*e*) The patient is unsteady and stands with his feet wide apart. His body and head may shake uncontrollably (titubation).

(*f*) Gait is staggering and broad-based.

(*g*) Muscle tone is reduced. The tendon reflexes are diminished and may be pendular.

Muscle tone

Tone is the resistance to the passive stretching of a muscle. It is dependent upon the physical properties of the joints, muscles and tendons, and the *muscle stretch reflex.*

Fig. 5 represents a voluntary muscle (M) with bony insertions at

AA. The muscle spindle (S) is arranged in parallel with the muscle (M) and is sensitive to changes in length.

If the points AA are drawn apart, the muscle (M) is stretched. Sensory impulses from the muscle spindle travel in the afferent nerve to the spinal cord where there is a single synapse with the motor cells of the anterior horn. The efferent limb of this reflex is via the alpha (fast conducting) motor nerve to the muscle (M). Thus, the muscle (M) contracts reflexly, pulling the points AA back to their original position.

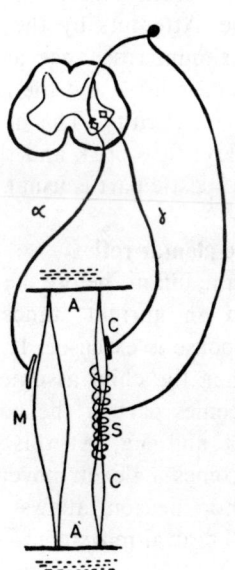

Fig. 5. The stretch reflex.
A—A Bony insertions of voluntary muscle M.
   C Intrafusal muscle fibre.
   S Muscle spindle.
   α Alpha (fast-conducting) motor nerve.
   γ Gamma (slow-conducting) motor nerve.

This is a cord reflex which if given free play would prevent any voluntary movement or change of posture. In health, supraspinal influences acting through pyramidal and extrapyramidal tracts modify this reflex. The descending fibres synapse with gamma motor nerve cells in the anterior horn. These slow conducting nerves activate the fine muscle strands CC which vary the length of the spindle receptor S. If the fibres CC contract, the muscle spindle is lengthened, there is a barrage of afferent impulses and the muscle (M) contracts reflexly. The points A—A are brought closer together.

Although the gamma system adapts slowly, it allows for fine, continuous adjustment of muscle action. Such a precise adjusting mechanism is appropriate for maintaining balance, for delicate manipulation and for homing on a target. It is unsuited to wide ranging, ballistic movements. Provision is made for isolating the gamma system and allowing the alpha system full control. Switching from gamma to alpha control and back, is a function of the extrapyramidal system. The 'switching mechanism' is probably sited in the cerebellum, but there is evidence that it also becomes disturbed in parkinsonism.

Interruption of the upper motor neuron releases the stretch reflex from cerebral influence. This causes a spastic increase in tone. Attempts by the examiner to overcome *spasticity* meet the maximum resistance at the beginning of the movement. There is then a release and the latter part of the movement is achieved with little difficulty. This is the clasp knife phenomenon. The tendon reflexes are brisk and the plantar responses extensor. Weakness of the spastic part is usual.

The plantar reflex
In the infant, before myelination of the nervous system is complete, and an upright stance has been achieved, the normal plantar response is extensor. It is part of the withdrawal response to pain. When the child assumes an upright posture, the plantar response becomes part of the postural reflex maintaining the tonus of the foot and leg. At this time the normal response to stimulation becomes a flexor movement of the toes. Interruption of the upper motor neuron allows the response to revert to the primitive withdrawal movement—the pathological extensor plantar.

Rigidity presents resistance throughout the range of passive movement. It is dependent upon an intact stretch reflex, but no clasp knife phenomenon is found. The resistance may be smooth—so called plastic rigidity or intermittent—cogwheel rigidity. Rigidity is a feature of disorders of the basal ganglia, and results from persistent gamma activity, and imperfect relaxation of the antagonist muscles. The muscle power and the tendon reflexes are not primarily affected. However, persistent contraction of the antagonists may make it impossible to elicit the tendon reflexes, and the patient fatigues rapidly in attempting to move his limbs against constant resistance.

Decrease in tone (hypotonia) is due to an interruption in either limb of the stretch reflex (p. 16), primary disease of the muscle or a lesion in the cerebellum. The affected part is flaccid, the tendon reflexes are diminished and the plantar responses, if present, are flexor.

Interruption of the stretch reflex causes recognizable weakness or loss of proprioception. Primary disease of the muscle gives rise to weakness and a clinical presentation described on page 196. Cerebellar disorders are accompanied by ataxia (p. 16).

Chapter 2
Sensation

An initial analysis of crude sensation is made at the periphery by the specialized sensory receptors. Light touch, pain, hot and cold sensation (temperature) and muscle/joint sense may thus be distinguished. Some of the special receptors are not found in many areas of the body, yet there is a normal sensitivity to the different sensory stimuli. Thus, the reception of the various forms of cutaneous sensation is not entirely dependent upon the specialized receptors.

Any peripheral stimulus is likely to activate several sensory nerve endings. It is the spatio-temporal pattern of neuronal activation in the spinal cord which determines and maintains the distinction between the different forms of sensation.

A lesion of the peripheral nerve usually causes loss of all forms of sensation, although a partial lesion often causes a more profound diminution of pain sensation.

Paraesthesiae are spontaneous sensations, often of a pricking or tingling nature. They are symptoms of neural irritation and are not experienced where denervation is complete.

Dysaesthesiae are abnormal, sometimes painful, sensations in response to stimuli. They are a variety of paraesthesiae.

A lesion of a peripheral nerve or posterior nerve root may be recognized by the distinctive area of sensory loss (Figs 6 and 7).

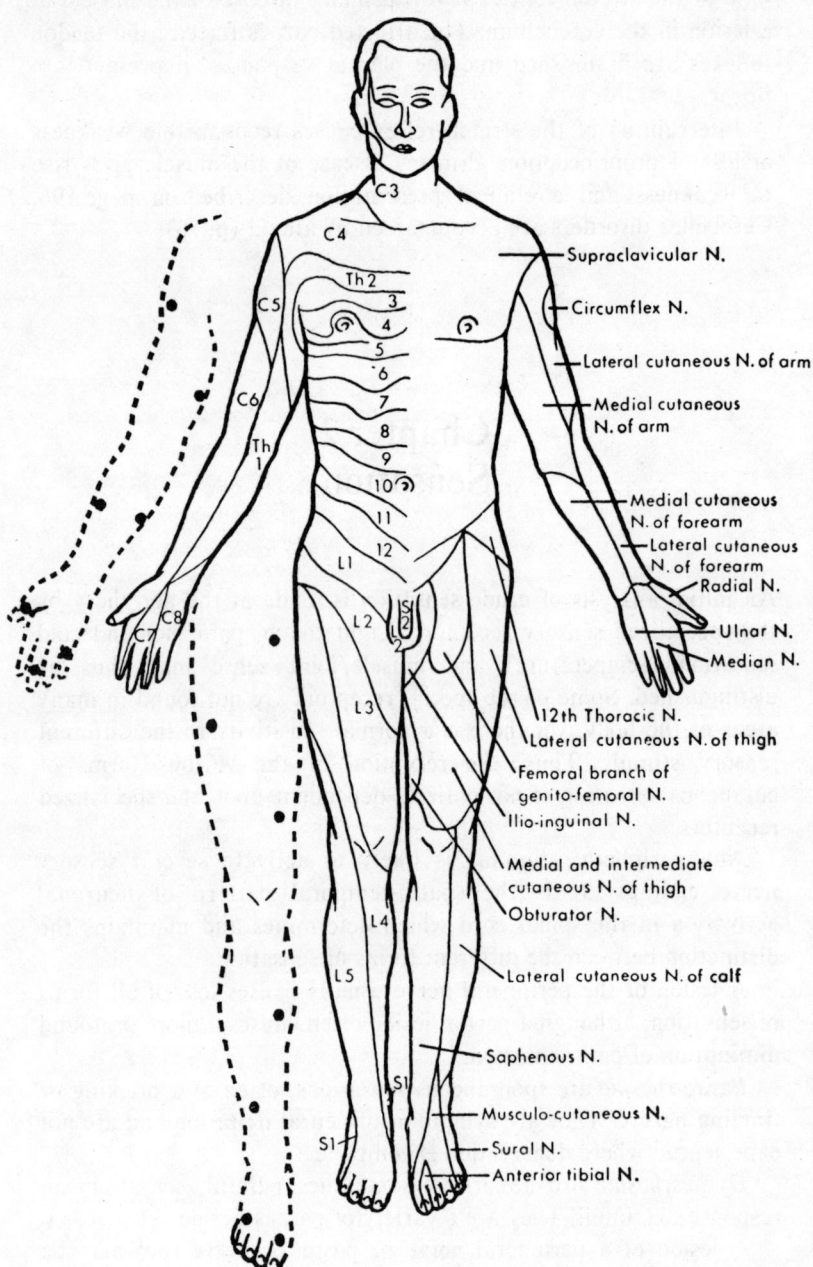

After entering the cord, the fibres subserving the different modalities regroup and join the appropriate ascending nerve bundles (Fig. 8).

Those carrying muscle/joint sensation, vibration and some touch fibres, enter the ipsilateral posterior columns without any intermediary synapse.

The other fibres synapse with cells in the posterior horn. These second order neurons give rise to fibres which cross in the anterior commissure of the cord, and join the contralateral spinothalamic tracts. These carry sensations of pain, hot and cold, and the rest of the light touch. Incomplete lesions of the spinal cord give rise to dissociated sensory loss (Fig. 8).

At the lower end of the medulla the fibres in the posterior columns synapse with their second order neurons in the cuneate and gracile nuclei. They then cross as the internal arcuate fibres to form the medial lemniscus (Fig. 19). This remains close to the mid-line until in the pons it begins to take a more lateral position, joining again with the spinothalamic tract (Figs 19–21). Both groups then synapse with thalamic nuclei. In the thalamus the sensory impulses are further organized before relay to the sensory cortex. Lesions in the thalamus raise the sensory threshold, but once this threshold is exceeded, the sensation is peculiarly unpleasant (thalamic syndrome). There is probably some crude appreciation of sensation at this level.

The sensory cortex which occupies the post-central gyrus (Fig. 1) has a somatic representation comparable with the motor cortex. Here localization and further analysis of the quality of sensation occur. Sensory loss resulting from a cortical lesion involves a functional unit such as a hand or a leg.

The interpretation of sensation is completed in the *parietal cortex*. Different modalities of sensation are correlated. Three dimensional images are formed, comparisons are made with previous experience, and association with the special senses and emotions collated. Lesions in the parietal cortex give rise to a distinctive clinical syndrome which is described on page 46.

Fig. 6 (facing page). Segmental and peripheral nerve innervation and points for testing cutaneous sensation of limbs (anterior). By applying stimuli at the points marked within the dotted outline, both dermatomal and main peripheral nerve distribution are covered simultaneously.

John Macleod, ed. (1964) *Clinical Examination*. Edinburgh and London. Churchill Livingstone.

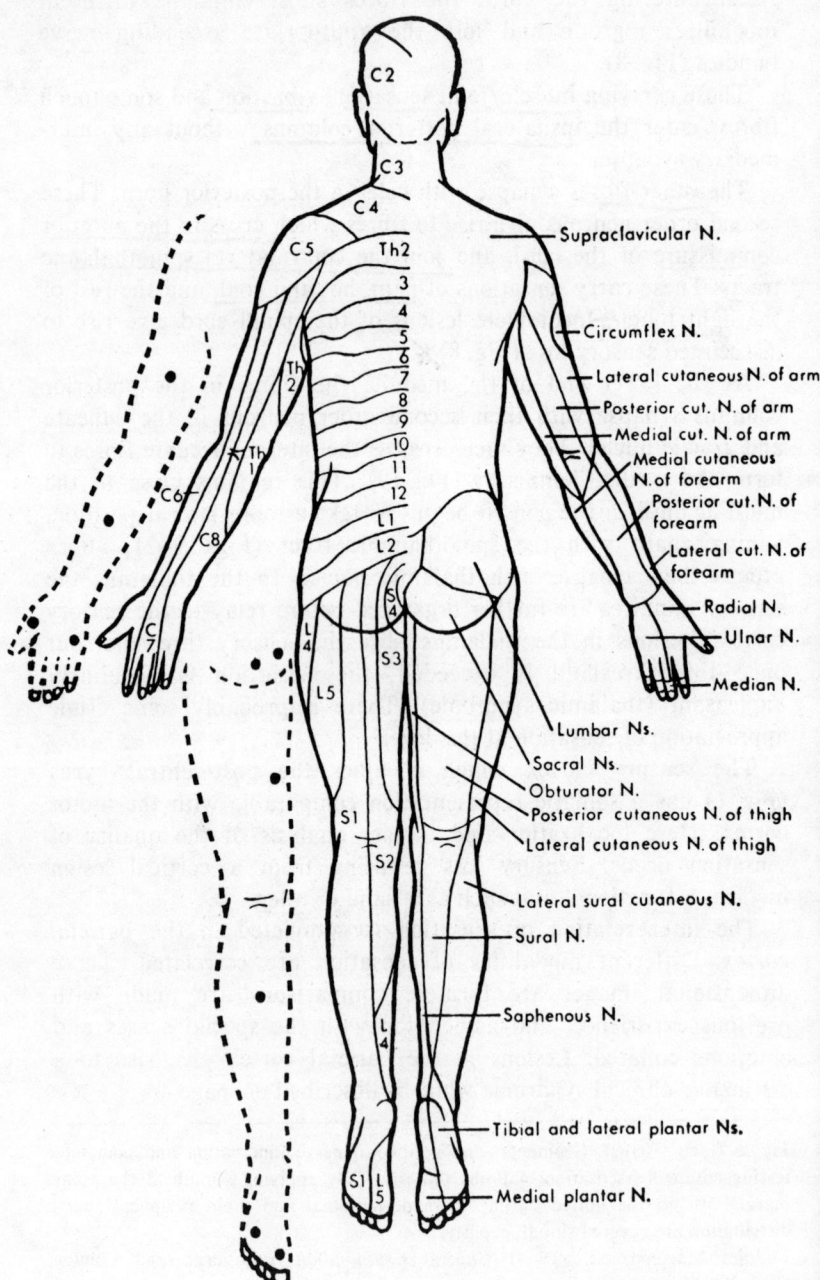

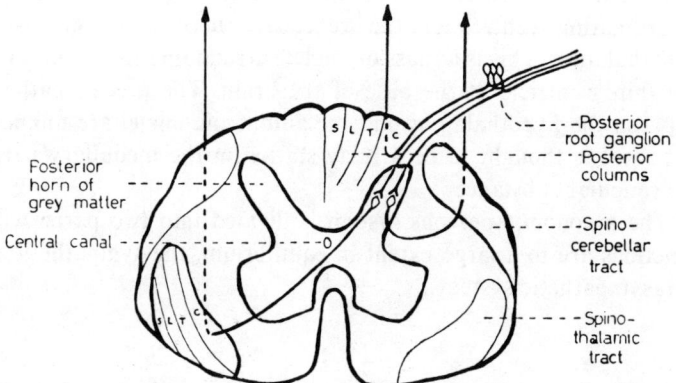

Fig. 8. Sensory nerve tracts in the spinal cord in the cervical region, showing decussation and the relative positions of fibres from the S. sacral, L. lumbar, T. thoracic and C. cervical roots.
Adapted from Bing.

Chapter 3
The Autonomic Nervous System

The role of the autonomic nervous system is to adjust the vegetative and visceral functions of the body to maintain a constant internal milieu. Its peripheral nerves supply the smooth (unstriated) muscle of the bronchioles, gut, glands, blood vessels, bladder and the heart. It is closely integrated with the metabolic and endocrine systems and although influenced by the individual's

---

Fig. 7 (facing page). Segmental and peripheral nerve innervation and points for testing cutaneous sensation of limbs (posterior). By applying stimuli at the points marked within the dotted outline, both dermatomal and main peripheral nerve distribution are covered simultaneously.

John Macleod, ed. (1964) *Clinical Examination.* Edinburgh and London. Churchill Livingstone.

emotional state it is outside his voluntary control. The chief co-ordinating centre for the vegetative nervous system is the hypothalamus. This is a mass of nuclei surrounding the lower part of the third ventricle at the base of the brain. The precise pathways between the hypothalamus and the autonomic nuclei are unknown, but there is thought to be a relay station in the medullary part of the reticular substance.

The autonomic nervous system is divided into two parts, whose functions are to a large extent in equilibrium, the sympathetic and parasympathetic systems.

THE SYMPATHETIC SYSTEM

The sympathetic nerves originate in the thoracic and upper two lumbar segments of the cord. In contrast with the somatic nervous system, the sympathetic (and parasympathetic) efferent impulses reach their target organs along a two-neuron chain. The cell bodies of the first or pre-ganglionic neurons lie in the lateral columns of the grey matter of the spinal cord. The sympathetic efferent fibres emerge in association with the somatic efferent fibres in the anterior nerve root. They then separate from the spinal nerve as the white ramus (Fig. 9). This terminates in one of the sympathetic ganglia which form a chain on the anterolateral aspect of the vertebral bodies from T1 to L2. The majority of fibres synapse here with the second neuron which reaches its destination either along a blood vessel or by rejoining one of the adjacent spinal nerves as the grey ramus. Afferent fibres return to the cord by the white ramus and the posterior nerve root.

With the exception of those fibres supplying the sweat glands, sympathetic neuro-somatic transmission is effected by the release of adrenaline. Sympathetic stimulation prepares the body for emergency action; the heart rate increases, the bronchioles dilate, blood is diverted from the skin to the muscles, the pupils widen and the subject breaks out in a sweat. Unlike the other sympathetic nerves, the sudo-motor fibres release acetylcholine at their post-ganglionic endings.

Interruption of the sympathetic supply to the skin gives rise to trophic changes. The skin becomes shiny, red and dry. The nails become beaked and cuts heal slowly.

The Autonomic Nervous System

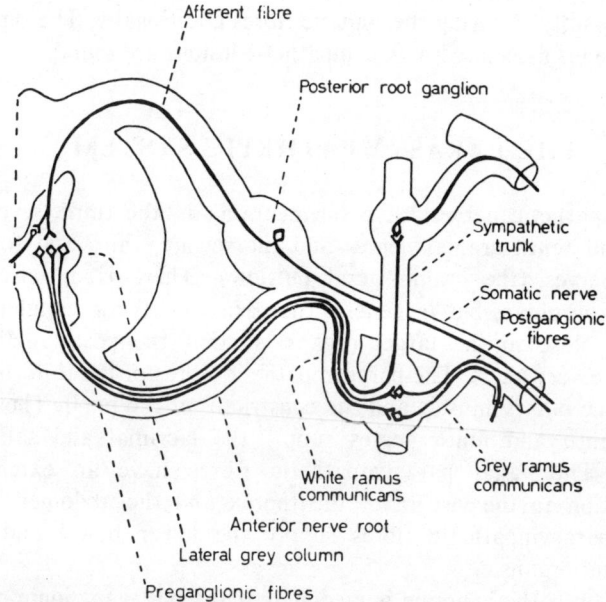

Fig. 9. Sympathetic nerve fibres, showing the relationships of the sympathetic trunk and spinal nerves and the dispersion of fibres over adjacent segments.
After Bailey and Cunningham.

Horner's syndrome

The sympathetic fibres which supply the head, emerge from the cord in the first and sometimes the second thoracic nerves, and ascend in the neck as the cervical sympathetic trunk. From the cervical ganglia, branches accompany the internal carotid artery into the cranium.

A lesion involving any part of this pathway, or the supraspinal sympathetic neurons in the lower brain-stem and cervical cord, results in the development of a Horner's syndrome. This consists of constriction of the pupil (meiosis), ptosis, apparent enophthalmos and the cessation of sweating over that side of the face (anhydrosis).

Causalgia is a particularly unpleasant and intractable pain following injury to a peripheral nerve. It most frequently involves the hand. The initial injury to the nerve is usually incomplete and affects both somatic and sympathetic fibres. This allows a short circuit of nerve impulses between efferent and afferent autonomic fibres possibly involving the somatic fibres additionally. The typical skin changes associated with sympathetic lesions are found.

THE PARASYMPATHETIC SYSTEM

Parasympathetic nerves leave the neuraxix in the third, seventh, ninth and tenth cranial nerves and the second, third and fourth sacral nerves (the cranio-sacral outflow). There is an efferent two-neuron chain, but in general the parasympathetic ganglia are situated close to the target organs, so that the post-ganglionic fibres are very short. The parasympathetic fibres of the third nerve supply the ciliary muscle and the constrictor of the pupil. Those of the seventh and ninth nerves supply the lacrimal and salivary glands. The vagal parasympathetic fibres have an extensive distribution to the viscera of the thorax and the abdomen. The sacral parasympathetic fibres supply the lower bowel and the urogenital organs.

Parasympathetic action is mediated at the post-ganglionic nerve endings by acetylcholine. It stimulates those functions of the body which are most appropriate to times of relaxation: digestion, bladder and bowel emptying, and sexual function. Blood is diverted from the muscle to the gut and the heart rate is slowed.

Referred pain
Autonomic afferent fibres from the viscera carry pain sensation to the spinal cord. These reach consciousness in company with the afferent somatic fibres from the same segment. Conscious interpretation of these stimuli is that the pain also originates externally, e.g. visceral afferent fibres from the heart accompany the mid cervical somatic nerves; thus, cardiac pain is referred to the shoulders and the left arm. Counter irritation at the site of the referred pain may block the original sensation.

BLADDER

The bladder wall is composed of smooth muscle innervated by parasympathetic nerve fibres arising in the second, third and fourth sacral segments of the cord. The parasympathetic nerves also carry afferent impulses. There is thus an autonomic reflex arc which causes the bladder wall to contract in response to distension of the bladder. The external sphincter of the bladder is, however, subordinate to supraspinal influences so that it is possible to inhibit the spontaneous (reflex) emptying of the bladder. The fibres concerned with voluntary control lie close to the pyramidal tracts in the cord. They synapse with the motor nerve cells of the first three sacral segments and emerge as the pudendal nerve which supplies the external sphincter. Sympathetic fibres from the lower thoracic and upper lumbar segments supply the bladder through the hypogastric plexus. The significance of the sympathetic efferent fibres is in doubt. The afferent fibres carry sensations of pain and fullness.

When the intravesical pressure rises to about 25 cm of water, afferent impulses from the bladder wall stretch receptors initiate mild rhythmical contractions of the detrusor muscles. A feeling of fullness reaches consciousness. Voiding begins with voluntary relaxation of the perineal muscles and the external sphincter. Bladder emptying is achieved by contraction of its muscle wall under control of the parasympathetic nerves.

Cystometry

Disordered bladder function is best studied by cystometry (Fig. 10). The patient is catheterized, using a catheter with a double lumen. Measured quantities of water are slowly introduced through one lumen, while the other is attached to a water manometer and an overflow. As water is introduced the intravesical pressure rises. A lengthening reaction in the muscle fibres of the bladder wall then occurs to accommodate the increasing volume and the pressure falls again. When 400–500 ml have been introduced, the intravesical pressure rises rapidly, the subject has the desire to void, and the bladder is emptied.

The atonic bladder

This is caused by interruption of either the sensory or the motor nerves to the bladder. There is an initial retention of urine while the bladder overfills. At the limit of the bladder walls' elasticity, overflow incontinence occurs. The atonic bladder has a large capacity, sometimes as much as five pints. With sensory lesions, e.g. tabes dorsalis, the patient has no feeling of fullness. Lesions of

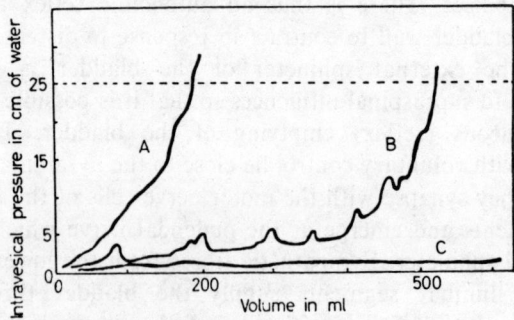

Fig. 10. Cystometrogam. Examples of recordings from:
  A. The reflex bladder.
  B. Normal bladder.
  C. Atonic bladder.

the anterior horn cells of the sacral cord cause overfilling which gives rise to intense pain and reflex hypertension.

The reflex bladder

This occurs with lesions of the spinal cord above the sacral segments, e.g. cord compression or disseminated sclerosis. Filling the bladder causes a constant rise in pressure without any relaxation. Emptying occurs after a small volume of water has been introduced, or sooner if muscular spasm is induced by stimulating the legs. The reflex bladder is generally small. If it is neglected its capacity may diminish to only a few ounces.

Incomplete cord lesions cause urgency, frequency or hesitancy of micturition.

Chapter 4
Cranial Nerves

I. THE OLFACTORY NERVE

The olfactory nerves are primitive outgrowths from the brain, lying in the olfactory groove in the floor of the anterior fossa. Central connections are made with the rhinencephalon (the smell brain), whose cortical representation, the olfactory tubercles lie on the underside of the cerebral hemispheres.

The sense of smell and sense of taste are closely linked and the olfactory nerve is responsible for one's appreciation of flavour. The sense of taste carried by the seventh and ninth nerves is limited to sourness, sweetness, bitterness and saltiness.

Anosmia is most commonly due to local disease in the nose, but may be caused by meningioma of the olfactory groove or fractures through the base of the skull.

II. THE OPTIC NERVE

Normal vision is dependent upon the physical properties of the cornea and lens; the co-ordinated action of the extraocular muscles, and the state of the retina. These are all available for direct examination. The neurology of vision concerns the optic nerves, the chiasm, the optic tract and lateral geniculate body, the optic radiation and the occipital cortex.

Light from objects in the temporal visual field falls on the nasal half of the retina, and light from the upper half of the visual field reaches the lower half of the retina. Optic nerve fibres are grouped into bundles as they leave the retina and pass through the cribriform plate of the optic disc. A rough, topographic orientation of these fibres is maintained as the nerve runs medially to the optic chiasm. Here, those fibres derived from the nasal half of the retina (the temporal visual field) decussate, while the fibres from the temporal half of the retina remain uncrossed (Fig. 11). Thus, the right optic tract is composed of fibres from the right half of each retina which 'see' the left half of both visual fields.

Fibres of the optic tract have three destinations:

(*a*) Lateral geniculate body—the majority of the fibres relay here to the optic radiation and cortex.

(*b*) The third nerve nucleus for pupillary light reflexes.

(*c*) Corpora quadrigemina—the reflex centre for the co-ordinated movement of head and eyes.

The uppermost fibres of the optic radiation pass directly backwards on the inferior surface of the parietal lobe round the posterior horn of the lateral ventricles to the visual cortex (Fig. 11). The lower fibres loop downwards and forwards in the temporal lobe around the inferior horn of the lateral ventricle and so to the visual cortex. As the spatial orientation of fibres is maintained from retina to cortex those fibres originating in the upper part of the retina form the direct upper fibres of the optic radiation, and vice versa.

The visual cortex occupies the area adjacent to the calcarine fissure on the medial and posterior aspects of the occipital lobe. The area of central (macular) vision has extensive cortical representation and a dual blood supply from the middle and posterior cerebral arteries.

Lesions of the visual pathway (Fig. 11)

A. *Optic nerve.* The visual disorder is limited to the affected side. A complete lesion causes total uniocular blindness. The direct pupillary response to light is lost, but the consensual response is retained. Pressure on the nerve or inflammation (optic neuritis) first affects the macular fibres resulting in a central scotoma.

B. *Optic chiasm.* Central lesions, such as a pituitary tumour, interrupt the decussating fibres and cause bitemporal hemianopia.

A laterally placed lesion, such as an aneurysm of the internal carotid artery, may cause a unilateral nasal hemianopia by compression of the non-decussating temporal fibres.

C. *Optic tract.* The close grouping of the fibres in the optic tract usually results in a complete, symmetrical hemianopia, without macular sparing. Careful use of a narrow beam torch may

Cranial Nerves

demonstrate the failure of the light reflex from the hemianopic area.

D. *Optic radiation.* As the fibres of the optic radiation become more dispersed, complete hemianopic lesions are less common.

Parietal lobe lesions involve the upper fibres causing lower quadrant field defects. Temporal lobe lesions involve the lower, indirect fibres causing upper quadrant field defects. The defects are usually congruous and there is no macular sparing.

The pupillary light reflexes are retained even from the blind part of the visual field.

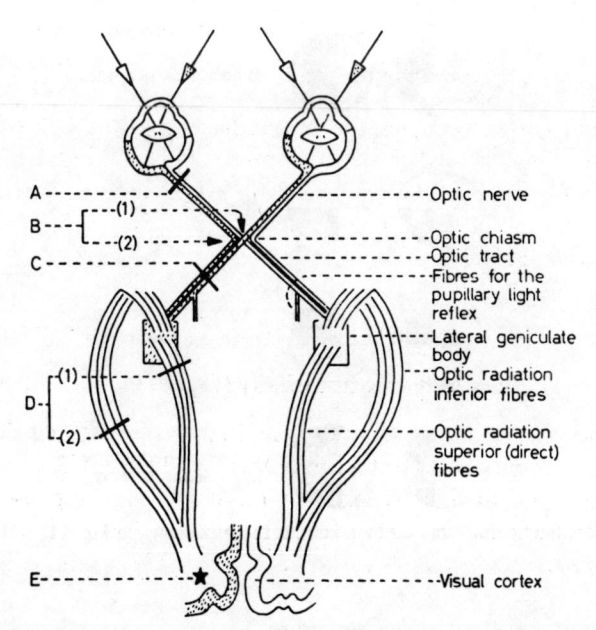

Fig. 11. The visual pathways showing the site of lesions causing characteristic field defects. See Fig. 11(a).

E. *Visual cortex.* Lesions of the visual cortex give rise to strictly congruous field defects. The central (macular) vision has an extensive cortical representation and may escape total destruction in a circumscribed lesion. It is also protected to some extent from the effects of ischaemia by the rich anastomosis between the posterior and middle cerebral arteries.

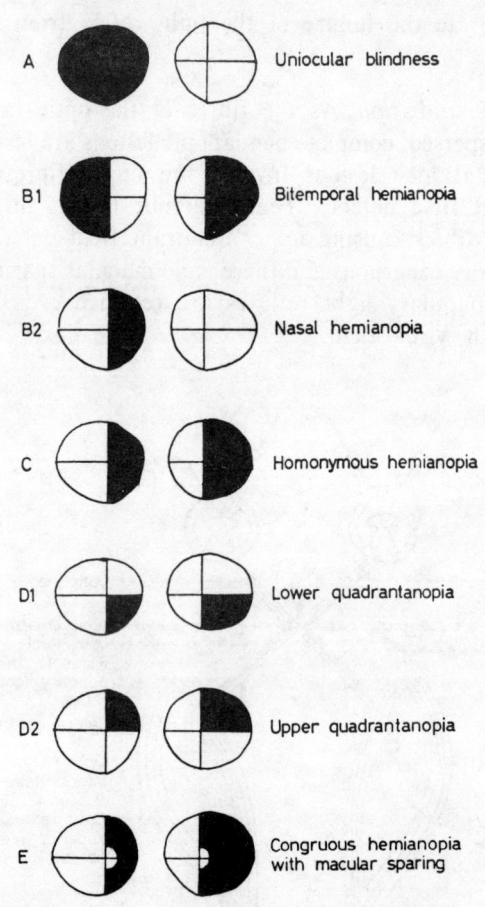

A — Uniocular blindness
B1 — Bitemporal hemianopia
B2 — Nasal hemianopia
C — Homonymous hemianopia
D1 — Lower quadrantanopia
D2 — Upper quadrantanopia
E — Congruous hemianopia with macular sparing

Fig. 11a. Visual field defects caused by lesions at the sites shown in Fig. 11.

Papilloedema—swelling of the optic disc.
The earliest signs of papilloedema are engorgement of the retinal veins, reddening of the disc, and blurring of the disc margins. As the swelling increases, the vessels become buried where they cross the raised disc edge. The swollen disc is then a dull purple in colour and the surrounding retina is streaked with haemorrhages.

The causes of papilloedema:
1. Obstruction of the venous outflow from the orbit. This is caused by raised intracranial pressure or thrombosis of the central vein of the retina or the cavernous sinus.

2. Inflammation of the optic nerve, e.g. optic neuritis.
3. Disease of the retinal vessels, e.g. malignant hypertension.

Optic atrophy
The atrophic disc has a dead-white appearance and a distinct margin. It is the late consequence of preceding disease which may or may not have been recognized.
The cause of optic atrophy:
1. Inflammation of the optic nerve.
2. Following papilloedema.
3. Familial neurological disorder, e.g. hereditary ataxia.
4. Head injury.
5. Systemic poisons, e.g. methyl alcohol.
6. Neurosyphilis.
7. Compression of the optic nerve, e.g. by tumour.
8. Vitamin B12 deficiency.
9. Retinal ischaemia due to prolonged or severe hypotension—often a result of haemorrhage.

(III, IV, VI) THE OCULOMOTOR, TROCHLEAR AND ABDUCENS NERVES

The nuclei of the third and fourth nerves lie in the upper mid-brain ventral to the aqueduct. The sixth nerve nucleus is in the lower pons, below the floor of the fourth ventricle. The nuclei lie in close relation to the medial longitudinal fasciculus which links them and the centres for conjugate eye movements (Fig. 16). Conjugate eye movement is under both voluntary and reflex control. The voluntary centre is probably in the precentral motor cortex. Stimulation of this area causes conjugate deviation of the eye towards the opposite side. The macula centring mechanism and the vestibular nuclei are the chief reflex controls. The third nerve supplies the levator of the upper eyelid, and all the extraocular muscles apart from the superior oblique (IV) and the lateral rectus (VI).

The nerves and muscles responsible for movements of the eye from the neutral position are shown in Fig. 12. When the eye is turned medially, downward movements are achieved by the superior oblique (IV) and elevation by the inferior oblique (III).

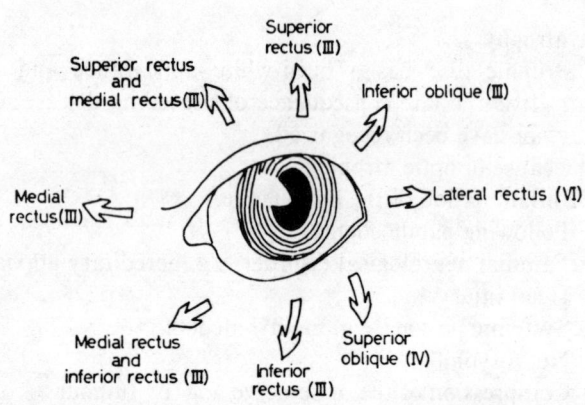

Fig. 12. The left eye showing the muscles and nerves responsible for movement of the eye from the neutral position.

Parasympathetic fibres arise in the Edinger–Westphal nucleus and travel in the third nerve to the ciliary ganglion. From here post-ganglionic fibres supply the sphincter of the pupil and the circular fibres of the ciliary muscle.

The central nucleus of Perlia provides supplementary innervation to both internal rectus muscles for the purpose of convergence, and in conjunction with fibres from the Edinger–Westphal nucleus supplies the sphincters of the pupils.

Light reflex

Shining a bright light into either eye normally results in prompt constriction of both pupils. The afferent fibres of this reflex leave the optic tract before reaching the lateral geniculate body. There is an intermediate synapse in the pretectal region of the mid-brain; from here fibres pass to the Edinger–Westphal nuclei on both sides. The efferent limb of the reflex travels by the third nerve to the ciliary ganglion and to the constrictor of the pupil. The crossing of fibres from the pretectal centre to both Edinger–Westphal nuclei accounts for the consensual light reaction.

A failure of the pupil to respond directly to light may be due to a lesion in the afferent pathway (optic nerve) or in the efferent pathway (IIIrd nerve). In the case of an optic nerve lesion the pupil will respond consensually to a light shone into the other eye. If it is due to a third nerve lesion, there is no direct response to light, but a consensual response in the other eye will be seen.

Convergence reflex
Where the individual fixes his gaze on a nearby object he converges his eyes and his pupils constrict. The afferent pathway of this reflex is probably from the visual cortex to the centres for conjugate eye movement in the precentral cortex, and from there to the central nucleus of Perlia. Fibres from the nucleus of Perlia supply both internal rectus muscles and by an ill-defined connection with the Edinger–Westphal nucleus supply the sphincters of the pupils. There is no relay of these efferent fibres in the ciliary ganglion, as there is for the light reflex, but there is probably a further synapse within the orbit.

Supranuclear palsies due to mid-brain tumour, brain-stem encephalitis, or cerebrovascular disease, cause paralysis of conjugate movement, either lateral or vertical.

Nuclear palsies of the third nerve are seldom complete, due to the dispersion of the individual nuclei in the brain-stem.

Third nerve lesions sometimes result from its entrapment by herniation of the temporal lobe through the tentorial opening, or from it stretched by an aneurysm of the posterior cerebral artery.

Lateral rectus palsy commonly accompanies raised intracranial pressure. The sixth nerve has an uncommonly long intracranial course where it is exposed to compression and traction.
  Muscle weakness which does not correspond to any particular nerve may be the result of myasthenia gravis, or ocular myopathy.

Argyll Robertson pupils are small and irregular in shape. They respond to convergence but not to light. Much the commonest cause is neurosyphilis. There is an interruption in the afferent limb of the light reflex between the point where the fibres leave the optic tract and where they synapse with the Edinger–Westphal nucleus.

Holmes–Adie syndrome
In this condition the pupils react very slowly to light and convergence. Relaxation of the pupils is similarly slow. Deep tendon reflexes may be absent. The WR is negative.

Strabismus (squint)
A gross inequality in the visual acuity of the two eyes, if present from an early age, may give rise to *concomitant strabismus.* The child does not learn to fuse the two visual images and does not achieve binocular vision. In concomitant strabismus, the angle of divergence of the ocular axes remains constant wherever the gaze is directed. When either eye is covered, the uncovered eye performs a full range of movements. The image from the weaker eye is suppressed and the patient does not have double vision. Concomitant strabismus may be prevented if suitable spectacles are used as soon as the defect is recognized.

Diplopia results from weakness of the extraocular muscles, occurring after binocular vision has been achieved. The two images diverge most widely when the eye is turned in the direction controlled by the affected muscle—*paralytic strabismus.*

Nystagmus

Nystagmus is a rhythmical oscillatory movement of the eyes resulting from a disorder of co-ordinated eye movement and fixation. It may be described as pendular, when the swings of eye movement are of equal velocity, or jerking when there are distinct fast and slow phases of movement. With the gaze fixed in one direction there is a slow drift of the eyes back to the neutral position and then a rapid correcting movement. Nystagmus is described as being in the direction of the fast movement. Jerk nystagmus is characteristic of cerebellar and vestibular disease while pendular nystagmus is due to defects in ocular fixation. The nystagmic movements can be horizontal, vertical or rotatory. The severity of nystagmus may be of three degrees.

First-degree nystagmus is seen only when the patient looks in the direction of the quick phase of the movement. Second-degree nystagmus is seen when the eye is in the neutral position, but is more exaggerated when the patient looks in the direction of the quick phase. Third-degree nystagmus is, in addition, seen when the patient looks in the direction of the slow phase.

Optokinetic nystagmus is a normal response of the eyes following objects moving past the visual fields.

Vestibular nystagmus
Rhythmical, often influenced by head movement and associated with vertigo.

Cerebellar nystagmus
Coarse, jerky movements. If the lesion is in the cerebellar hemisphere the nystagmus is most prominent on looking towards the side of the lesion. Intoxication with barbiturates, phenytoin or alcohol causes a cerebellar type of nystagmus.

Retinal nystagmus
Miner's nystagmus. A result of working in light which is too dim for effective macular vision. This causes defective retinal fixation with a consequent pendular nystagmus.

Congenital nystagmus
Defective vision in early life causes a pendular nystagmus.

Brain-stem nystagmus
Involvement of the medial longitudinal fasciculus in brain-stem disorders, e.g. disseminated sclerosis, causes nystagmus associated with defects of conjugate eye movement. It is often uniocular.

(V) TRIGEMINAL NERVE

The trigeminal nerve supplies, by its three divisions, common sensation to the face and scalp as far back as the vertex (Fig. 13). It also supplies the mucous membrane of the sinuses, the nose, mouth, tongue and the teeth. The motor root innervates the muscles of mastication; the masseters and pterygoids. Proprioceptive fibres from these muscles travel in the mandibular division of the nerve. The trigeminal (sensory) ganglion lies in a pouch of dura on the surface of the petrous part of the temporal bone. The two roots enter the brain-stem on the ventral surface of the pons (Fig. 20).

The fibres carrying touch sensation terminate in the main sensory nucleus soon after entering the brain-stem. The second order neurons cross the midline and join the medial lemniscus on its way to the thalamus. The fibres carrying pain and temperature sensation pass down the brain-stem as the spinal tract of the fifth nerve. One by one they enter the spinal nucleus of the fifth nerve which extends into the upper cervical cord. The second order neurons decussate and join the spinothalamic tract. Unlike the peripheral divisions of the fifth nerve, the spinal nucleus retains the primitive segmental representation. Pain sensitive fibres from the muzzle area of the face enter the nucleus first, followed by those from the surrounding areas of the face (Fig. 14). Fibres from in front of the ear descend as far as the second cervical segment. Thus a lesion in the cervical cord may give rise to a ring of facial analgesia.

Fig. 13. The peripheral divisions of the trigeminal nerve. Oph. Ophthalmic or first division. Max. maxillary or second division. Mand. mandibular or third division.

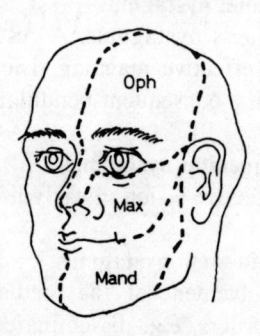

The proprioceptive fibres terminate in the mesencephalic tract of the fifth nerve, which extends from the main sensory nucleus into the midbrain on the lateral aspect of the periaqueductal grey matter.

Jaw jerk
The afferent limb of this reflex is carried by the proprioceptive fibres in the mandibular division and the efferent limb by the motor root of the trigeminal nerve. An increased jaw jerk is indicative of an upper motor neuron lesion above the level of the pons.

Glabellar tap
This is a reflex elicited by tapping rhythmically on the root of the

nose. The afferent pathway is by the ophthalmic division and the efferent path by the facial (VII) nerve. The blink reflex is normally supressed after the first few taps, but it persists in parkinsonism.

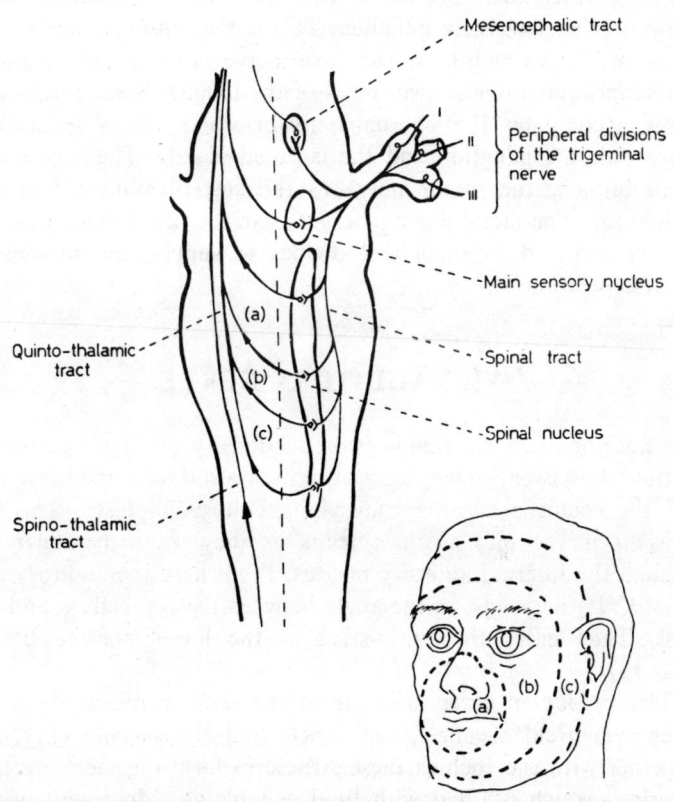

Fig. 14. The central connections of the trigeminal nerve. The fibres of the spinal tract and nucleus retain the primitive segmental relationship. Showing the extent of analgesia caused by lesions at (a)—(c).

(VII) FACIAL NERVE

The facial nerve has motor, sensory and autonomic divisions. The sensory and parasympathetic fibres form the intermediate nerve of Wrisberg. The facial motor nucleus lies deep in the lower pons. Its fibres first pass dorsally to encircle the sixth nerve nucleus before emerging with the intermediate nerve in the cerebello-pontine angle (Fig. 19). The fibres conveying taste sensation terminate in the tractus solitarius.

With the acoustic nerve (VIII) they enter the internal auditory meatus and then pass into the facial canal.

Within the canal the motor root and the intermediate nerve merge in the geniculate ganglion. This is the sensory ganglion for the taste fibres which leave the facial nerve as the chorda tympani and supply the anterior two-thirds of the tongue. Some autonomic fibres accompany the chorda tympani while others go to the sphenopalatine ganglion and the lacrimal glands. There is also a small branch, the motor nerve to the stapedius muscle of the middle ear. The facial nerve emerges from the facial canal through the stylomastoid foramen and divides to supply the muscles of facial expression.

(VIII) AUDITORY NERVE

The auditory nerve contains two functionally different parts, the vestibular division, conveying postural sensation from the labyrinth, and the cochlear division conveying auditory impulses. The two divisions merge into a single trunk as they leave the inner ear through the internal auditory meatus. From here the auditory and facial (VII) nerves lie in the angle between the cerebellum and the pons. They enter the brain-stem at the lower pontine border (Fig. 19).

The *vestibular nerve* arises from the sensory receptors in the three semicircular canals, the utricle and the saccule (Fig. 15). Together with the cochlea these structures form the membraneous labyrinth which is filled with fluid endolymph. Movement of the head stimulates the nerve endings in the ampullae of the semicircular canals. By virtue of the spatial arrangement, movement in any plane causes inertial displacement of endolymph. The canals are thus sensitive to acceleration and direction of movement. The utricle contains small granules supported on hair-like processes. These respond to the absolute position of the head and linear movements. The function of the saccule is unknown.

In the pons, most of the fibres of the vestibular nerve terminate in four vestibular nuclei, while a few pass directly to the cerebellum. Fibres emerging from the vestibular nuclei have three main destinations (Fig. 16).

Cranial Nerves

1. The motor nuclei of the spinal cord, via the vestibulo-spinal tract. These form part of the postural reflex arc.
2. The cortex of the temporal lobe. These serve the conscious appreciation of equilibrium.
3. The medial longitudinal fasciculus, and so make connections with:

(a) the centre for conjugate eye movement and the nuclei of the third, fourth and sixth cranial nerves;
(b) the palaeocerebellum, which smoothes the vestibular stimuli and relays them to the extrapyramidal system for correcting movements;
(c) the motor nuclei of the neck muscles;
(d) the reticular formation.

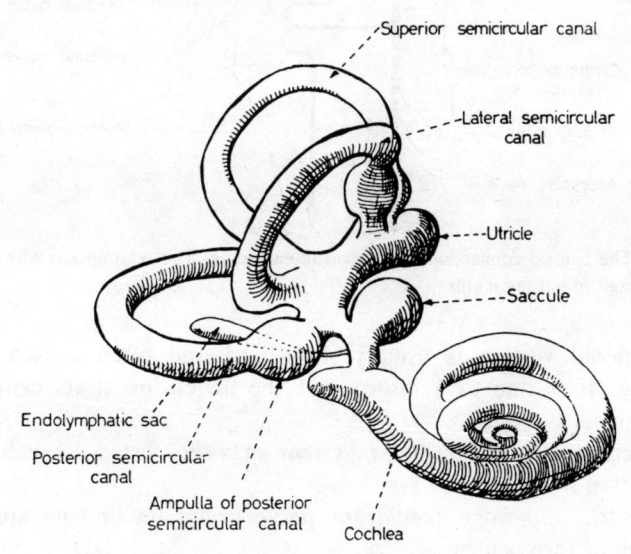

Fig. 15. The membraneous labyrinth of the right side seen from the right.

A sense of equilibrium depends upon a continuous and balanced flow of impulses from the two sides. **Vertigo** is caused by failure of one or both vestibular systems. Vertigo is an unpleasant sense of motion, affecting the individual or his environment. It is usually rotatory so that objects seem to spin round, or it may be vertical so that the ground appears to tilt. A gradual unilateral failure may go unnoticed by the patient until he is subjected to some extreme postural disturbance. Sudden failure provokes severe vertigo, often making the patient fall but there is no loss of consciousness. He is nauseated, pale and sweating. Examination reveals rhythmical nystagmus, with the fast component away from the affected side.

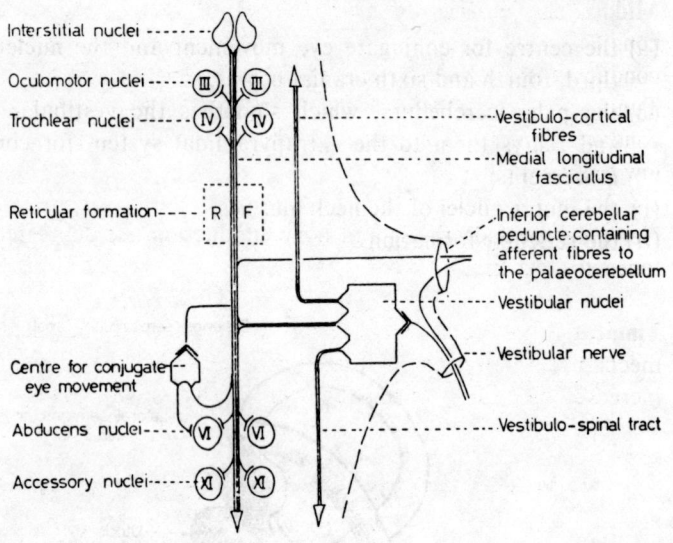

Fig. 16. The central connections of the vestibular nerve. The relationship with the medial longitudinal fasciculus.

Positional vertigo is usually short-lived and often caused by stooping. It is due to a disorder of the utricle or of its central connections.

Function of the vestibular system may be tested by caloric stimulation (p. 72).

The true *auditory (cochlear) nerve* originates in the spiral ganglion of the cochlea.

Sound travels by air conduction along the external auditory canal to the tympanic membrane. Three jointed ossicles transmit and amplify a mechanical stimulus across the middle ear to the oval window, and so to the endolymph of the cochlea. The spirally arranged organ of Corti lying within the cochlea makes the initial separation of sound into tones before it is transmitted along the nerve. The auditory nuclei are laterally placed beneath the floor of the fourth ventricle. Fibres from the auditory nuclei decussate as the corpus trapezoideum and then form the lateral lemniscus which passes up the brain stem in company with the medial lemniscus. There is a relay station in the medial geniculate body; from here fibres continue to the auditory cortex on the superior aspect of the temporal lobe.

Middle ear deafness is due to a disorder of the mechanical conduction of sound received at the tympanic membrane. Sound conducted direct to the inner ear through the skull is not affected. Tuning fork tests show that air condition is depressed while bone conduction remains normal. Middle ear deafness causes a loss of low tones first.

Nerve deafness. Both air and bone conduction are depressed. High tones are lost first.

Tinnitus is a persistent hissing or buzzing sound, caused by mechanical irritation, by partial lesions of the nerve, or by increased blood flow in the adjacent internal carotid artery.

(IX, X) GLOSSOPHARYNGEAL AND VAGUS NERVES

These can be considered together as they form a functional unit, share the same medullary nuclei, run a similar course, and are often both involved by a single lesion.

Their motor fibres originate in the nucleus ambiguus, those of the ninth going to the stylopharyngeus and the tenth to the voluntary muscles of the larynx and pharnyx.

Their sensory fibres terminate in the nucleus solitarius. Those of the ninth supply common sensation to the nasopharynx and posterior aspects of the soft palate and tongue, and taste fibres to the posterior third of the tongue. The sensory fibres of the tenth supply the thoracic and upper abdominal viscera and a small area in the external auditory canal. The parasympathetic fibres of the ninth supply the salivary glands while those of the tenth innervate the viscera. The ninth, tenth and eleventh cranial nerves leave the skull by the jugular foramen. Isolated lesions of the ninth and tenth nerves are uncommon and both are usually implicated in posterior fossa tumours, or fracture of the base of the skull. The recurrent laryngeal branch of the vagus is sometimes involved in thoracic disease when paralysis of the vocal cords and dysphonia result.

(XI) SPINAL ACCESSORY NERVE

This is a motor nerve with cranial and spinal fibres. The cranial fibres originate in the nucleus ambiguus like those of the ninth and tenth. The spinal contribution is from the upper cervical segments. It innervates the upper fibres of the trapezius and the sternomastoid. There is a contribution to the muscles of the larynx.

(XII) HYPOGLOSSAL NERVE

The hypoglossal nerve is the motor supply to the muscles of the tongue. Its nucleus is the medullary homologue of the spinal anterior horn cells. Unilateral lesions cause the tongue to be deviated towards the side of the lesion.

Lower motor neuron lesions give rise to atrophy of the tongue and fasciculation. The fasciculations are seen as continuous fine wriggling movements beneath the mucous membrane.

Chapter 5
Functional Topography of the Brain

Certain areas of the brain have specific functions, and discrete lesions cause comparable disabilities. The most important divisions are shown in Fig. 1, but no attempt has been made to illustrate the subcortical connections or the commissures connecting the two hemispheres. These are important in that a lesion involving the subcortical connections may give rise to symptoms which are referable to a distant part of the cortex.

In general, the right hemisphere receives sensation from, and controls the movement of, the left side of the body.

However, upper motor neuron fibres from both hemispheres innervate the muscles of the upper part of the face, jaw, neck and trunk, preserving these movements in the presence of hemiplegia.

Irritative lesions cause positive symptoms referable to areas shown in Fig. 1. Thus, a Jacksonian motor seizure may result from a scar on the motor cortex. Destructive lesions cause a loss of function, for example, infarction of the occipital lobe causes hemianopia.

The prefrontal cortex is termed a silent area as there is little knowledge of its function. There are, however, specific clinical signs which point to disease in this area. These are:

Mental change—the patient is likely to be apathetic, forgetful and careless of his personal condition, particularly if the disease involves both frontal lobes.

The grasp reflex—if the examiner draws his finger across the patient's palm, it will be grasped firmly. It can be elicited in the stuporous patient and, if unilateral, is highly suggestive of a contralateral frontal lesion.

Ataxia—the ataxia of frontal lobe lesions may be indistinguishable from cerebellar ataxia. It is thought to be due to an interruption of the pathway between the motor area, basal ganglia and cerebellum. It is sometimes accompanied by akinesia.

Motor cortex
Destructive lesions cause contralateral upper motor neuron weakness. Irritative lesions cause focal motor or Jacksonian motor seizures. Jacksonian seizures are typified by spreading clonic jerks, e.g. from the thumb to the fingers, to the hand, to the forearm and arm. The irritative process spreads from a focus on the cortex along the precentral gyrus. The thumb, a corner of the mouth, or the great toe, are frequent points of origin. Lesions between the two hemispheres involve both legs and sometimes the bladder.

Accessory motor cortex
This lies anterior to the cortical motor representation for the lower limb, on the medial surface of the hemisphere (Fig. 1). Irritative lesions in the accessory motor cortex give rise to tonic postural movements of the head and limbs.

Sensory cortex
Irritative lesions of the sensory cortex give rise to contralateral paraesthesiae which may be localized or spreading in the same way as the similarly caused symptoms in the adjacent motor cortex. Destruction causes loss of sensation.

Parietal lobe
This extensive area of the brain cannot be related to specific parts of the body. Rather it is responsible for the interpretation and correlation of sensation. There may be any form of sensory loss but astereognosis and diminished two point discrimination are outstanding.

Astereognosis (tactile agnosia). This is a difficulty in recognizing the size, weight, texture and shape of an object by touch alone.

Two point discrimination. This tests the patient's ability to recognize simultaneous but spatially separate stimuli. The normal individual can distinguish the two points of a pair of dividers only 2 or 3 mm apart when they are pressed on to the pulp of his finger. The accuracy varies from individual to individual and over different parts of the body. The most significant finding is a difference between the two sides of the body.

Sensory suppression may be found. If stimuli are applied simultaneously to both sides of the body, the sensation is neglected on the side contralateral to the affected parietal lobe.

The patient may experience temporal and geographic disorientation, so that he loses his way when in a normally familiar neighbourhood or even inside his own house.

Two well-delineated syndromes are associated with parietal lobe lesions, Gerstmann's syndrome and disorders of body image.

Gerstmann's syndrome is found only with lesions of the dominant hemisphere. It consists of right/left disorientation, inability to recognize the individual fingers, defective calculation and agraphia.

Disorders of the body image accompany lesions of the non-dominant hemisphere. The individual may neglect an otherwise useful limb, deny ownership of a limb, and fail to recognize the disability of a paralysed limb.

Parietal lobe lesions sometimes cause muscular atrophy, and if in the dominant hemisphere, disorders of consciously organized movements, apraxia (p. 11).

Functional Topography of the Brain

Occipital lobe—visual cortex
Irritative lesions may cause crude visual sensations—such as flashes of lights in the contralateral half field. Destructive lesions cause visual field defects (p. 31).

Temporal lobe
Those parts of the cerebral cortex directly concerned with taste, smell and hearing are situated in the temporal lobe. In addition, it is responsible for the organization of memory, and it has close functional connections with the association areas of the visual cortex and somatic sensory cortex. It is intimately connected with the hypothalamus and so with the visceral motor system and the physical control of emotions.

Disease of the temporal lobe gives rise to characteristic disorders of memory, hallucinations of smell, taste, sight and sound; behavioural anomalies, and in the dominant hemisphere, dysphasia. These symptoms are particularly prominent as a result of irritative lesions—that is, in temporal lobe epilepsy (p. 91). Destructive lesions cause less easily recognizable symptoms. An expanding lesion will often invade the optic radiation, causing an upper quadrantic field cut (Fig. 11).

Brain-stem
Three nuclear masses lie embedded in the white matter of the cerebral cortex at the upper end of the brain-stem. These are the thalamus, the basal ganglia and the hypothalamus (Fig. 4). They form the primitive head nuclei and organizing centres of the sensory, motor and autonomic systems respectively. From here the afferent and efferent conducting pathways extend down through the mid-brain, pons and medulla oblongata to the spinal cord. The brain-stem also contains the nuclei of cranial nerves III to XII, the cerebellar pathways and the reticular formation. The reticular formation is a network of nuclei and connecting fibres, responsible for the motor and sensory relays, the control of the vital centres, and the mechanism for cortical arousal.

Thalamic lesions raise the threshold of peripheral sensation. However, once this new threshold is exceeded, painful stimuli provoke a diffuse, burning reaction. This is the thalamic syndrome. Disease of the basal ganglia causes rigidity, bradykinesia and involuntary movements. Lesions involving the hypothalamus cause disorders of thirst, appetite, growth and temperature regulation.

Chapter 5

Familiarity with a simplified anatomy of the brain-stem is required for the localization of lesions at this site. The sections (Fig. 18–21) show the relative positions of the main fibre tracts and nuclei. It should be noted that the structure of all four sections is basically the same if the areas below the broken lines are discounted.

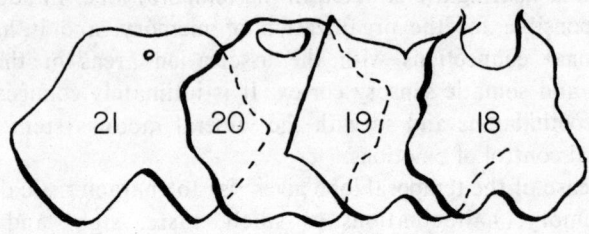

Fig. 17. Orientation of the brain-stem sections in Figs 18–21.

1. *The medial longitudinal fasciculus* is constant in it position close to the mid-line below the floor of the aqueduct and the fourth ventricle.
2. The *spinothalamic tract* maintains its lateral position but moves dorsally in the higher sections.
3. As the *medial lemniscus* ascends through the brain-stem, it is displaced laterally from its original mid-line position in the lower medulla.
4. The *cranial nerve nuclei.* There are no simple rules which order the siting of the cranial nerve nuclei. The position of certain

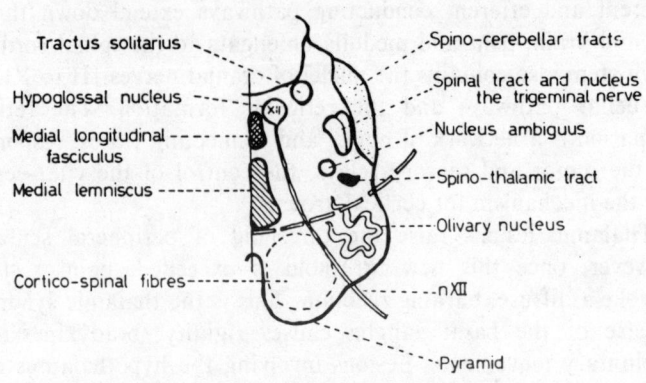

Fig. 18. Section through the medulla. After Buchanan.

key nuclei is helpful in locating brain-stem lesions. The nuclei of the third and fourth nerves in the midbrain, the sixth nerve in the pons and the twelfth nerve in the medulla, lie in the grey matter beneath the floor of the aqueduct and fourth ventricle.

The nucleus ambiguus is an elongated motor nucleus serving the ninth, tenth and eleventh nerves. This with the motor nuclei of the fifth and seventh nerves in the pons form a broken column placed deeper and more laterally in the brain-stem.

The sensory nuclei of the fifth and eighth nerves occupy lateral positions in the pons. The spinal tract and nucleus of the fifth nerve extend caudally to the second cervical segment of the cord.

5. The areas below the broken lines contain the *descending corticospinal fibres*. In the midbrain they form large cohesive nerve trunks, the basis pedunculi. These are the direct downward

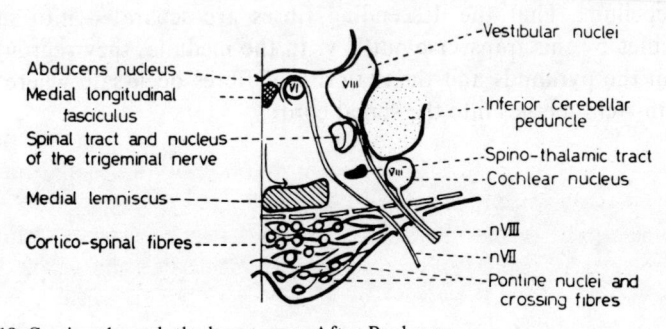

Fig. 19. Section through the lower pons. After Buchanan.

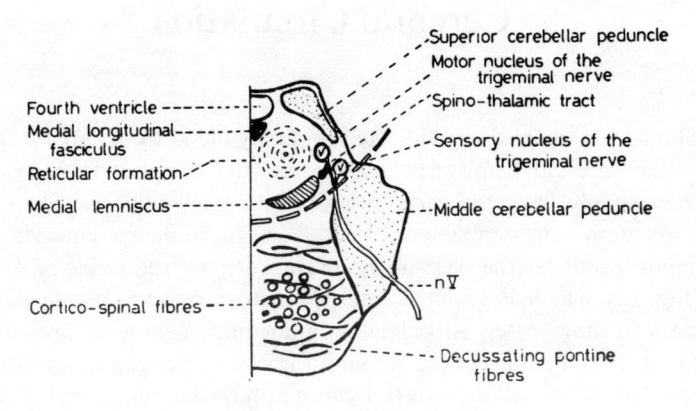

Fig. 20. Section through the mid-pons. After Buchanan.

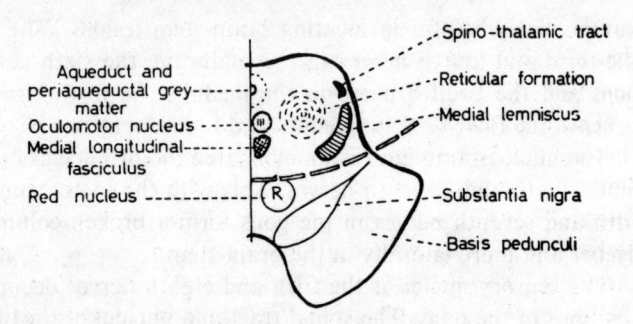

Fig. 21. Section through the midbrain. After Buchanan.

projections from the internal capsules. In the pons, some of these fibres synapse with the pontine nuclei and the second-order neurons stream across the mid-line to form the middle peduncles of the cerebellum. Thus the descending fibres are separated into small bundles by this transverse outflow. In the medulla, they regroup to form the pyramids and the majority of fibres decussate where the brain-stem merges into the spinal cord.

Chapter 6
Cerebral Circulation

The paired internal carotid arteries supply blood to the greater part of the cerebral hemispheres. However, the occipital lobe gets its chief supply from the vertebrobasilar system which also feeds the brain-stem and cerebellum. There are anastomoses between the major vessels at the base of the brain, forming the *circle of Willis* (Fig. 22) which lies in the interpeduncular cistern. If one of the main feeding vessels is occluded, an adequate collateral circulation can usually be established through the circle. Congenital atresia or absence of one of the arteries can similarly be compensated. The occurrence of degenerative vascular disease at a later date then

Cerebral Circulation

causes more extensive brain damage than might otherwise be expected. The circle of Willis and its immediate branches are common sites for aneurysms.

The *common carotid artery* divides at the upper border of the thyroid cartilage to give the external and internal carotid arteries. Immediately beyond its origin is a common site for stenosis of the *internal carotid artery*. The artery enters the skull through the petrous part of the temporal bone and then makes a double curve through the cavernous sinus. Here there is an important branch, the ophthalmic artery, which supplies the retina. Leaving the cavernous sinus, the internal carotid pierces the dura and the arachnoid, and gives off the posterior communicating artery and the anterior choroidal artery. This contributes to the supply of the basal ganglia, thalamus and internal capsule. The internal carotid artery then divides into the anterior and middle cerebral arteries.

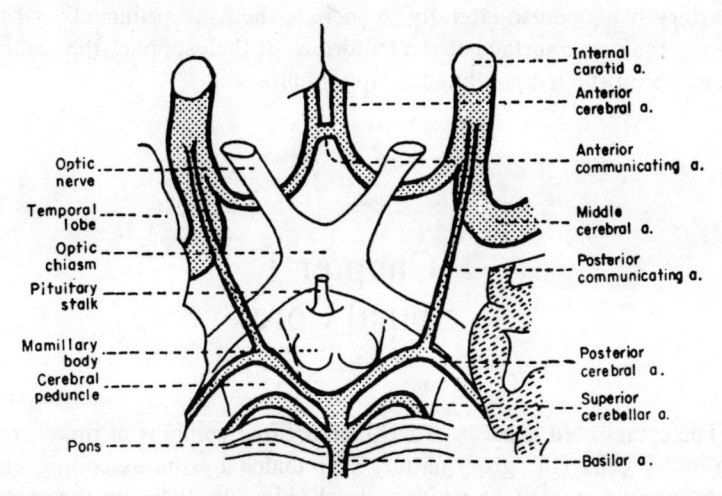

Fig. 22. The circle of Willis and its relationship with the base of the brain, seen from below.

The *anterior cerebral artery* proceeds towards the mid-line and rises between the two hemispheres. There is a small anterior communicating artery between the anterior cerebral arteries of the two sides. The medial striate artery is an important branch which also supplies the anterior half of the internal capsule. With this exception the territory of the anterior cerebral artery is limited to the medial aspect of the hemispheres.

The *middle cerebral artery* gives off several small branches. The lateral striate arteries supply the basal ganglia and internal capsule. It then passes laterally through the Sylvian fissure where it divides into its terminal branches. These branches extend over the surface of the hemisphere.

In the neck the slender *vertebral arteries* ascend through the foramina in the transverse processes of the vertebrae. They enter the skull through the foramen magnum and join to form the basilar artery on the ventral surface of the pons. The posterior inferior cerebellar arteries are given off before the fusion. These supply the lateral part of the medulla and the cerebellum.

Paired vessels arise from the single *basilar artery*. The anterior inferior cerebellar arteries, the pontine arteries and the superior cerebellar arteries, have well-marked anastomoses. Occlusion of any one seldom causes symptoms. The basilar artery finally divides to form two posterior cerebral arteries. Each posterior cerebral artery swings dorso-laterally to encircle the basis pedunculi and to gain the upper surface of the tentorium. It then supplies the medial surface of the temporal and occipital lobes.

Chapter 7
Spinal Cord

The spinal cord consists of well-demarcated columns of motor and sensory cells (the grey matter) surrounded by the ascending and descending tracts (the white matter) (Fig. 23). It lies in the spinal canal and like the brain is surrounded by three fibrous membranes, the meninges. It is cushioned by the cerebrospinal fluid and held in place by the denticulate ligaments. Paired sensory and motor roots, corresponding to each segment of the cord, emerge from the canal by the intervertebral foramina. The cord segments are shorter than the corresponding vertebrae and the spinal cord terminates at the level of the first or second lumbar vertebra. The lowermost segments (sacral) are compressed into the last inch of the cord, known as the *conus medullaris*. The subarachnoid space extends

Spinal Cord

beyond the end of the cord as far as the second sacral vertebra. This space is traversed by the remaining nerve roots, the *cauda equina*. A lumbar puncture needle may be introduced into the subarachnoid space, below the level of the second lumbar vertebra, without any danger of damaging the spinal cord.

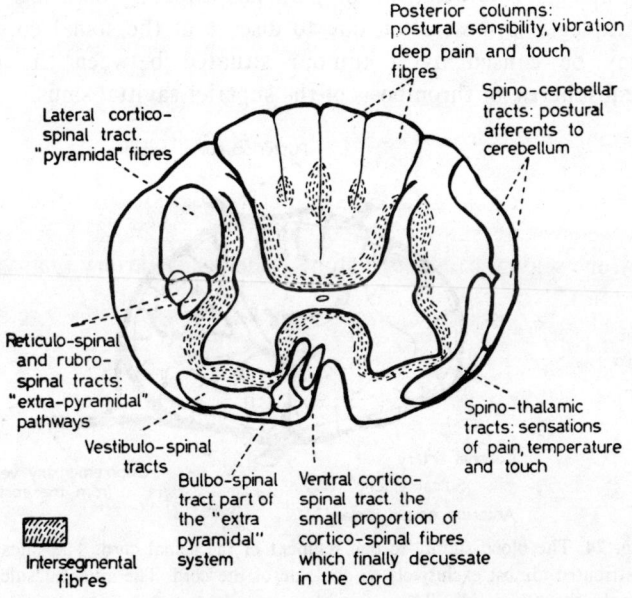

Fig. 23. The fibre tracts of the spinal cord. The short intersegmental fibres pass up and down and across the spinal cord, drawing adjacent segments into reflex activity. After Truex.

An *anterior and two posterior spinal arteries* extend along the length of the cord. They are branches of the vertebral arteries and are supplemented by auxiliary vessels from the aorta. The supplementary arteries enter the spinal canal through the intervertebral foramina. There are usually one or two cervical feeders, three thoracic and two lumbar. The anterior spinal artery gives off coronal branches which encircle the cord and anastomose with the small posterior spinal arteries. The tissue of the spinal cord derives its most important blood supply from the sulcal arteries which arise at intervals along the length of the anterior spinal artery (Fig. 24). Fine branches from the anastomotic ring supply the peripheral part of the cord. As can be seen from the diagram (Fig. 24), the posterior and lateral columns adjacent to the grey matter are least well supplied and so suffer first in ischaemic cord lesions.

Paraplegia

Paraplegia is a weakness or paralysis affecting both legs. Spastic paraplegia is most often due to disease of the spinal cord, but it may be caused by a tumour situated between the cerebral hemispheres, or thrombosis of the superior sagittal sinus.

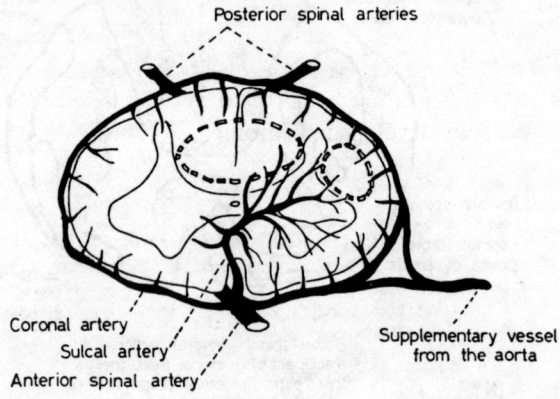

Fig. 24. The blood supply to one segment of the spinal cord. The sulcal artery is distributed almost exclusively to one side of the cord. The adjacent sulcal arteries supply the other side. There are also short branches passing in a longitudinal direction. The two 'watershed' areas at risk in ischaemic lesions are shown.

Interruption of the corticospinal tracts releases the reflex arcs of the cord from supraspinal inhibition. The tendon jerks are brisk and the plantar responses extensor. Any painful stimulus causes a flexion withdrawal of the legs. In this state of heightened excitability the mere touch of clothing is sufficient to provoke flexor spasms. If the reticulospinal pathways remain intact, postural reflexes will predominate so that extensor tone is heightened. Extensor tone will be enhanced by appropriate physiotherapy so that the paraplegic patient can support himself on his feet.

The paraplegia which results from an acute transverse cord lesion may at first be flaccid. This is the state of 'cord shock' and usually resolves after three to six weeks. A flaccid paraplegia will result from a compressive or destructive lesion of the cauda equina.

In addition to the paraplegia, there is commonly a loss of sensation and disordered bladder function below the level of the lesion. In the case of a cauda equina lesion, the sensory loss is in a saddle distribution.

The Brown-Séquard syndrome

A unilateral compressive or destructive spinal cord lesion may give rise to the Brown-Séquard syndrome. It is the result of a hemi-section of the cord and consists of ipsilateral cutaneous anaesthesia and lower motor neuron paralysis at the level. of the lesion, ipsilateral spastic paralysis and proprioceptive sensory loss below the level of the lesion, and contralateral loss of spinothalamic sensation below the level of the lesion. It is unusual to find the fully developed syndrome.

Chapter 8
Cerebrospinal Fluid

Cerebrospinal fluid (CSF) is formed by diffusion and active secretion from the choroid plexuses of the ventricles and from the vessels in the subarachnoid space. The different constituents are formed at different rates under normal and pathological conditions.

The main flow is from the lateral ventricles through the foramina of Monro to the third ventricle, along the aqueduct to the fourth ventricle and out to the subarachnoid space through the foramina of Magendie and Luschka. It bathes the pial surface of the cord and brain, penetrating deeply into the tissue of the nervous system, along the blood vessels.

There is a differential reabsorption of the constituents of the CSF. Some water and electrolytes are reabsorbed within the ventricles, although this may occur passively for the maintenance of ionic equilibrium. The greater part is absorbed into the venous circulation from the surface of the brain and spinal cord. The protein is reabsorbed into the arachnoid granulations along the venous sinuses within the skull and into the veins of the nerve root sheaths in the spinal canal.

Obstructions to the outflow of CSF at any point within the brain cause an internal hydrocephalus, with dilatation of the ventricles upstream of the obstruction. Communicating hydrocephalus is caused by interference with the absorption of the CSF. This may be due to thickening and adhesion of the meninges following meningitis or to thrombosis of the venous sinuses.

There is free and rapid passage of substances between the brain and the CSF, but there is a barrier between the blood and CSF, the blood–brain barrier. This maintains a constant milieu for brain metabolism and is a protection against noxious substances in the circulation. The barrier is equally effective against antibiotics except when inflammation changes its characteristics.

Cerebrospinal fluid may be examined by needling the subarachnoid space between lumbar vertebrae 3 and 4 or 4 and 5.

Normal CSF is clear and colourless. Its normal constituents are:

Protein: $0 \cdot 1 – 0 \cdot 5$ g l^{-1}
Glucose: $2 \cdot 5 – 4 \cdot 5$ mmol l^{-1}
Chloride: $118–125$ mmol l^{-1}
Cells: $0–5$ lymphocytes mm^{-3}

Dynamics: the pressure of the CSF should be measured before any fluid is withdrawn. The patient should be allowed to relax and lie quietly, breathing through his mouth. The normal resting pressure is between 50 mm and 150 mm of CSF. If there is any suspicion of spinal cord compression the Queckenstedt manoeuvre should be performed. An assistant compresses both sides of the patient's neck with the flat of his hands. This occludes the venous return from the brain raising the intracranial pressure. There is normally a brisk rise in the pressure of CSF which falls back to normal when the compression is released. Lesions which block the spinal canal prevent this transmitted rise in pressure.

The *colloidal gold curve* (Lange curve): abnormal globulin in the cerebrospinal fluid will precipitate gold from a colloidal suspension. The colloidal gold is put up in a series of tubes and increasing dilutions of cerebrospinal fluid are added. The degree of precipitation is graded from zero to five (complete). Normal CSF causes no precipitation. Maximum precipitation in the first tubes of the sequence is called a first-zone curve or paretic curve, e.g. 555431000, from a case of general paresis. Maximum precipitation in the middle tubes is called a mid-zone or tabetic curve, e.g.

Cerebrospinal Fluid

001344210, from a case of tabes dorsalis. Either may be found in disseminated sclerosis (p. 172). First zone curves are also found in the non-metastatic neurological complications of carcinoma (p. 203) and in subacute panencephalitis. The gamma globulin fraction can be measured directly and is expressed as a percentage of the total protein. More than 15 per cent is considered abnormal and 30 per cent would strongly support the diagnosis of a demyelinating disease or neurosyphilis.

Raised intracranial pressure

An increase in the volume of the intracranial contents results in a rise in pressure. This is compensated at first by a displacement of CSF and blood but a point is soon reached when the venous drainage is obstructed and the pressure then rises even more quickly.

The common causes of raised intracranial pressure
  1. An expanding lesion, such as a neoplasm or abscess, or due to haemorrhage in the brain substance, or in the subdural or extradural space.
  2. Oedema of the brain, due to trauma or inflammatory disease.
  3. Impaired absorption of CSF, e.g. thrombosis of venous sinuses.

The rising CSF pressure is transmitted to the subarachnoid space surrounding the optic nerves. Consequent compression of the central vein of the retina causes papilloedema.

Raised pressure due to a supratentorial lesion may cause herniation of the brain downwards through the tentorial opening and the foramen magnum. This results in compression of the mid-brain or medullary centres (coning). The abducens nerve may be trapped in its long course giving rise to diplopia or the herniating temporal lobe may compress the third nerve resulting in a dilated pupil.

The occurrence of progressive or fluctuant drowsiness, headache and vomiting should rouse the suspicion of increasing intracranial pressure. *In the presence of papilloedema, lumbar puncture should be avoided.* The removal of CSF may precipitate fatal coning.

Chapter 9
Consciousness

Consciousness is an individual's awareness of himself and his environment. It is dependent upon the inflow of information presented by the sensory nerves and special senses and its relay from the reticular formation in the brain-stem to the cerebral cortex. Consciousness is also dependent on the level of activity of this reticulo-cortical system. Conversely, unconsciousness results from hypofunction of the reticular activating system and consequent depression of cortical activity. Centres in the reticular formation maintain the cerebral cortex in a state of wakeful receptiveness.

Adequate nutrition (oxygen and glucose) is essential for the efficient functioning of the cortex and activating system. Nutrition is maintained by the rich cranial blood supply which constitutes more than 15 per cent of the cardiac output.

Sleep is a normal state of altered consciousness. This is achieved partly by a natural rhythmicity of the activating centre and partly by the withdrawal of external stimuli. In contrast to pathological unconsciousness an individual can easily be aroused from sleep.

Causes of altered consciousness
1. Head injury
2. Epilepsy.
3. Intoxication.
4. Vascular disease.
5. Infections.
6. Compressive lesions.
7. Metabolic disorders.

Head injury
Severe head injury causes a transient loss of consciousness—concussion. Shearing forces in the brain-stem or altered blood flow to the alerting centres may be responsible. More severe injuries cause swelling of the brain or compression of brain tissue by haemorrhage.

Epilepsy
A recurrent disorder characterized by altered cerebral function, usually with some degree of altered awareness. It may be a genetically determined disorder or a consequence of other diseases of the brain.

Intoxication
The ingestion of drugs or poisons having a direct depressant effect on the alerting centres of the brain stem and the cortex e.g., sedatives, tranquillizers, psychotropic drugs, alcohol, solvents.

Vascular disease
Reduced blood flow to the brain secondary to vascular disease or hypotension. Infarction. Haemorrhage due to degenerative vascular disease or aneurysm.

Infection
Meningitis or encephalitis. Cerebral abscess usually presents as a compressive lesion.

Compressive lesions
Space occupying lesions, such as tumour, abscess or haematoma raise the intracranial pressure having a direct effect on the centres for alertness in the brain-stem, and interferring with the normal circulation of blood and CSF. Herniation of the uncus through the tentorial opening aggravates the direct pressure on the upper brain-stem with deepening unconsciousness.

Metabolic disorders
Hypoglycaemia and diabetic ketoacedosis. Myxoedema and hypopituitarism. Renal and liver failure. Electrolyte imbalance and disorders of calcium metabolism.

Chapter 10
Higher Functions

The means by which the brain analyses and correlates incoming sensory stimuli, and responds to them. The response may be immediate, for example, a movement, or it may involve reference to memory and the establishment of new memories or the stimulus may provoke a spoken response.

In general the left hemisphere is the site of verbal activity and abstract reasoning; the functions underlying non-verbal responses, spatial awareness and perception are situated in the right hemisphere.

Speech
Verbal communication is closely related to reading, writing and gesture, and is necessary for most forms of abstract thought. Perception itself is influenced by the observer's language resources.

The development of fluent speech depends upon normal hearing, normal intelligence and the ability to produce co-ordinated movements of the mouth, tongue and larynx; less readily distinguishable by clinical examination, but equally important, is an intact system of subcortical association fibres between the parietal, sensory and motor areas of the cerebral cortex. A child usually acquires his first recognizable words at one year, and at two to two and a half years he is making short sentences. His understanding of language precedes his ability to express himself. Speech development may be delayed by emotional or social deprivation and juvenile psychoses.

The child who does not speak presents a complex problem of evaluation. Psychometry, audiometry, neurological assessment with special attention to parietal function, and a consideration of the family history and emotional environment will contribute to one's understanding of the problem and to the formulation of appropriate treatment.

A speech disorder which first manifests itself in adult life should be regarded as a symptom of a new disease process. If the disorder is one of articulation it is called dysarthria. If it is a defect in the use of language it is known as dysphasia. The terms dysphasia and aphasia are used interchangeably. Dysphasia may be primarily receptive or primarily expressive. Seldom are the two forms completely separable and mixed forms of dysphasia are common.

The patient with an expressive (motor) dysphasia has difficulty in expressing his thoughts by articulate sounds. He may be unable to find the appropriate word (nominal aphasia) or to enunciate polysyllabic words. In the more severe forms he is unable to make himself understood; his speech may be reduced to meaningless sounds or to an incomprehensible sequence of nominal and grammatical errors. In a lesser degree his speech may consist of isolated nouns and verbs without the usual inflexions and without the use of articles and conjunctions, resulting in a telegraphic style whose meaning is however clear. Expressive dysphasia is a disorder in the construction of language and may be likened to apraxia. The patient is frustrated and distressed by his disability.

Receptive (sensory) dysphasia interferes with the patient's comprehension of the spoken word. Minor degrees can be recognized by his failure to appreciate abstract concepts, for example the meaning of proverbs and figures of speech. The individual with severe receptive dysphasia cannot appreciate or act on instructions and his attempts to speak are marred by uncorrected mistakes (jargon aphasia). Receptive dysphasia is a defect in the analysis of language and is related to agnosia.

Recognition of the type of dysphasia is of limited value in locating the responsible lesion. In general the 'speech areas' of the brain are in the dominant left hemisphere, of a right-handed person. A lesion in the perisylvian region of the left hemisphere will usually cause some degree of dysphasia. A lesion in the non-dominant hemisphere of a right-handed person seldom gives rise to dysphasia. In left-handed subjects the speech areas are usually in the left hemisphere, but a lesion in the right hemisphere may also cause dysphasia. Expressive dysphasia results from a lesion in front of the lower end of the motor cortex. This is called Broca's area. Receptive dysphasia may be caused by lesions scattered over a wide area of the temporo-parietal lobes. In this situation an interruption of the subcortical association fibres is probably of more significance than the damage to the overlying cortex.

Memory

Learning is a process whereby an individual's behaviour is modified as a result of practice. This implies plasticity of neural function. Memory is the ability to store and retrieve learned material.

All of an individual's experiences register briefly in his short-term memory and unless they are consolidated they are dissipated within a few seconds. The physical concommitant of short-term memory is probably a transient electrochemical trace through the neurons involved.

In longer lasting memory, the neuronal trace is thought to involve a redistribution of the RNA and protein within the cells. More permanent memories require an activation of a neuronal chain through the temporal lobe, hippocampus, fornix and mammillary bodies. 'Memories' as such are probably the facilitated synaptic links between neurons in those parts of the brain which were originally activated by the remembered experience. Long-term memories are consolidated by repetition; the readiness with which consolidation occurs depends on the individual's motivation, alertness, and the emotional content and familiarity with the material involved.

Retrieval of remembered items requires a reactivation of the temporal hippocampal axis.

Pathological disorders of memory most commonly interfere with the registration and retention of new information. The patient presents with an amnesia for recent events with a relative sparing of more distant memories.

Disorders involving the thalamus, hypothalamus, mammillary bodies and the temporal lobe give rise to amnesia. Tumour, infarction, viral encephalitis, vitamin deficiency, trauma and electroconvulsive therapy may be responsible.

Part II
The History and Examination

The History and Examination

In the majority of cases a diagnosis can be made on the information contained in a carefully taken history. The precise nature, the extent and severity of the disease usually depend upon the result of the examination.

After taking the history from the patient, confirmation may be sought from members of his family, or from a witness to any specific episodes.

First, the patient should be allowed to give his own description of his complaints. The examiner should then attempt to clarify any ambiguous symptoms. Illness is often outside the patient's normal experience, and he may have difficulty in expressing his complaints. It should be remembered that seemingly specific medical terms often have quite different meanings to the patient. Persistent questioning may be necessary to elucidate the true meaning of such terms as dizziness, faintness, blackout, double vision, spasm and numbness. The patient should always be asked about the occurrence of headache, visual symptoms, deafness, vertigo, abnormalities of his sense of smell and taste, weakness and altered sensation in his arms and legs, bladder dysfunction and any alterations of consciousness.

An attempt should be made to establish the chronological pattern of the illness. The date on which symptoms developed and when there was improvement or relapse. It may be possible to establish some relationship with other events such as injury, pregnancy, climatic changes, etc.

The account should include details of the patient's birth, early development, previous health and any injuries. The occurrence of neurological disease, endocrine disturbance and mental illness in the family should be noted. Education, occupation, drinking habits, travel and possible exposure to venereal disease may be significant.

Examination
The examination of the nervous system is made within the context of the general physical examination. Neurological disease may be secondary to or co-exist with disease elsewhere in the body. Until considerable experience has been gained, a strictly methodical

scheme of examination should be followed. Although this may seem rather rigid it ensures that nothing is neglected. The precise order is unimportant, but the examination must include:
1. The head and cranial nerves.
2. The mental state and speech.
3. The neck and trunk.
4. Power, sensation, tone and co-ordination in the arms.
5. Power, sensation, tone and co-ordination in the legs.
6. Reflexes.
7. Stance and gait.

While taking the history an assessment can be made of the mental functions, including memory, mood and speech. During the general inspection particular attention should be paid to:

A. The head—its shape, any abnormal protuberance, or tenderness. The examiner should listen with his stethoscope over the carotid arteries and skull for any bruit.
B. Deformity of the spine or limbs.
C. Involuntary movements.
D. Muscle bulk—hypertrophy, wasting and fasciculation.
E. Pigmentary changes, including naevi and birthmarks.

Cranial Nerves

(I) Olfactory nerve
First ensure that the nasal passages are clear. Using some easily recognized aromatic substance such as orange, tobacco, or soap, each nostril is tested in turn. Ask the patient if he can smell anything and then whether he can identify it. Pungent substances should be avoided as they stimulate the trigeminal fibres in the nasal mucosa.

(II) Optic nerve

(a) *Acuity*
Both distant and near vision may be tested. In the routine examination it is sufficient to test near vision only, using a test card of standard type. Each eye is tested in turn, with and without spectacles if these are normally worn. The acuity is then expressed as the smallest size of type which can be read. If necessary, Snellen charts are used for distant vision.

(b) Visual fields

Confrontation. The patient and examiner sit facing each other at a distance of two feet. The patient covers his right eye and the examiner covers his left. The patient is told to look into the pupil of the examiner's eye while a small object such as the head of a hat pin (white) is brought into the visual fields from the periphery. The patient indicates when it first appears and the extent of his field is compared with the examiner's (normal) field. Several points on the periphery are tested in this way. The other eye is then tested. A permanent record of the peripheral fields can be made using perimetry. Defects in the central visual fields and the size of the blind spot can be mapped on the Bjerrum screen.

By noting the reaction to a feint, a rough idea of field size may be obtained in the uncooperative patient.

(c) Fundi

Examination of the fundus oculi is made with a hand ophthalmoscope. The patient is told to fix his gaze on a distant object. When examining the right eye, the observer should use his right eye and hold the ophthalmoscope in his right hand. If difficulty is experienced in seeing the fundus, the student may find it helpful to begin the examination at a distance of two feet from the patient. While looking through the eye-piece of the ophthalmoscope he gradually closes with the patient until the fundus comes into view. He should focus his attention, in turn, on the optic disc, the retina, the vessels and the macula.

The optic disc. The normal disc is creamy pink and its temporal margin is clearly seen. The nasal margin may merge with the retina, but it is not perceptibly raised. The centre of the disc is hollowed forming the optic cup and is paler in colour.

An abnormal disc may be atrophic or swollen. The atrophic disc is clearly demarcated from the retina and chalky-white in colour. The swollen disc is reddish-purple in colour, the edges are blurred and the centre may be obviously heaped up (papilloedema). Streaky haemorrhages are seen on the surface of the disc and the surrounding retina. The veins are distended and may be buried in the surface of the disc.

Retina. Note is made of the colour, the presence of haemorrhages and exudates, and atrophy of the choroid.

Vessels. The course of the four main arteries and their accompanying veins should be followed. Any aberrant or obstructed vessels are noted and the calibre of the veins is compared with that of the arteries. This is normally 3:2, but may be increased in raised intracranial pressure. Attention should be paid to the arterio-venous crossings. In hypertensive disease the walls of the arteries are thickened and rigid. This compresses the veins where the two cross (A-V nipping).

Macula. This is seen by asking the patient to look directly at the light of the ophthalmoscope. The macula is normally free from vessels and slightly darker than the surrounding retina. Degenerative changes are found in some of the inherited neurological disorders.

(III, IV, VI) Oculomotor, trochlear and abducens nerves

The third, fourth and sixth nerves are usually examined at the same time. When the eye is at rest in the neutral position, the muscles and nerves responsible for movement are those shown in Fig. 25. When the eye is turned medially, downward movement is performed by the superior oblique and elevation by the inferior oblique. Fourth nerve lesions are most easily demonstrated when the eye is turned inwards. There is then a failure of downward movement.

Imperfect function of one muscle or group of muscles may be so slight as to be inapparent to the examiner. The patient should be questioned regarding the occurrence of double vision (diplopia). To determine which muscle is involved, the examiner should move the test object to the position where the images are most widely separated. This will be the direction in which the affected muscle moves the eye. The patient should then identify the false image which is the outermost of the two, and is usually fainter. Covering the affected eye will extinguish the false image.

The full range of eye movements is tested and the width of the palpebral fissure measured. The pupillary reactions to convergence, and the direct and consensual pupillary reactions to light, are tested. The presence, direction and degree of nystagmus is noted.

(V) Trigeminal nerve

Light touch, pain and temperature sensation are tested on both sides of the face, in the three peripheral divisions. Pain sensation should also be tested round the nose and mouth, and on the periphery of the face to exclude involvement of the spinal nucleus of the fifth nerve in the lower brain-stem.

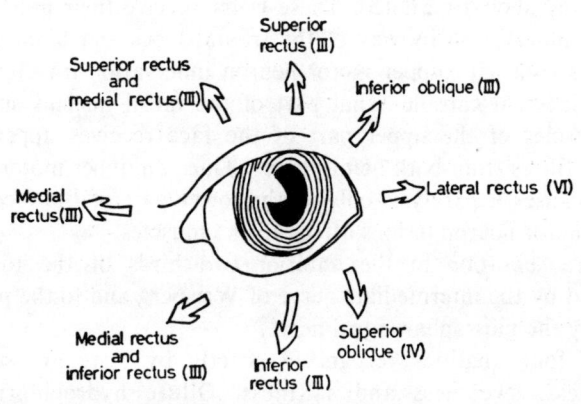

Fig. 25. The left eye showing the muscles and nerves responsible for movement of the eye from the neutral position.

The bulk of the temporalis and masseters may be assessed during inspection of the head. The power of jaw closure (masseters) and the opening and lateral movements of the jaw (pterygoids) should be tested. In unilateral lesions of the motor root, the jaw deviates towards the paralysed side.

The jaw jerk. The afferent limb of this reflex is carried by the mandibular division, and the efferent limb by the motor root of the fifth nerve. The patient is told to relax and let his mouth hang half-open. The examiner grasps the tip of the chin between his thumb and first finger and taps the top of his thumb with a tendon hammer. An increased jaw jerk results in the teeth snapping briskly together. It is often difficult to elicit in the normal individual. A brisk jaw jerk is evidence of a bilateral upper motor neuron lesion, above the level of the pons.

The corneal reflex. Touching the cornea with a wisp of cotton wool makes the patient blink with both eyes. Sensation from the cornea travels in the ophthalmic division of the trigeminal, and the efferent pathway depends on the facial nerves of both sides.

(VII) **Facial nerve**

Voluntary facial movement is tested by asking the patient to wrinkle up his brow and frown, to close his eyes tightly, to show his teeth in a wide smile, to purse his lips and puff out his cheeks.

While talking to the patient, spontaneous facial movements such as smiling should be noted. These latter receive their upper motor neuron innervation by way of the frontal lobes and basal ganglia, whereas voluntary upper motor neuron innervation travels by way of the internal capsule. That part of the facial nucleus supplying the muscles of the upper part of the face receives upper motor neuron fibres from both hemispheres. Thus, an upper motor neuron lesion causes a paralysis only of the lower part of the face, while lower motor neuron lesions affect all the muscles.

Taste sensation to the anterior two-thirds of the tongue is supplied by the intermediate nerve of Wrisberg and to the posterior third by the glossopharyngeal nerve.

The four qualities recognized strictly by taste are sourness, bitterness, sweetness and saltiness. Dilute hydrochloric acid, quinine sulphate, sugar and salt are used as test substances.

The patient should be allowed to wash out his mouth with clean water before and after each test. He is then told to put out his tongue and a small quantity of the substance is touched on it. He indicates to the examiner when he recognizes the taste and he is allowed to withdraw his tongue and identify the substance.

As can be seen from Fig. 26 the site of a facial nerve lesion can be determined with some accuracy from the combination of symptoms and signs.

(VIII) Auditory nerve

Tests of hearing. The external auditory canal should be examined to ensure its freedom from cerumen and for evidence of disease of the tympanic membrane. Testing each ear in turn, a note is made of the maximum distance at which the patient can hear a quiet whisper (normally this is more than three feet).

Diminished hearing may be due to a lesion of the cochlea and cochlear nerve (*nerve deafness*) or to a disorder of the mechanical conduction of sound in the middle ear (*conduction deafness*). The tuning fork tests are used to differentiate between nerve and conduction deafness. In the normal individual and in patients with nerve deafness, sound transmission by air and the ossicles of the middle ear is more efficient than transmission through the bone, and thus seems louder. Disease of the middle ear impairs the mechanical conduction of sound by the ossicles and so bone-conducted sound seems louder.

Rinne's test. A 512 cycle s^{-1} fork is struck and its base placed on the mastoid process, while the ear is occluded. The patient

The History and Examination 71

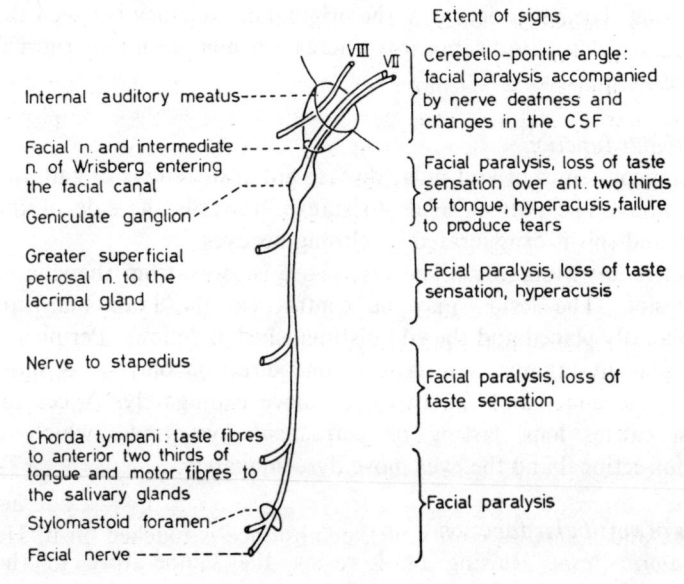

```
                                    Extent of signs
                          VIII  VII  ⎫ Cerebello-pontine angle:
Internal auditory meatus-----⟋        ⎬ facial paralysis accompanied
                                      ⎭ by nerve deafness and
Facial n. and intermediate              changes in the CSF
n. of Wrisberg entering              ⎫ Facial paralysis, loss of taste
the facial canal                     ⎬ sensation over ant. two thirds
Geniculate ganglion                  ⎭ of tongue, hyperacusis, failure
                                       to produce tears

Greater superficial                  ⎫ Facial paralysis, loss of taste
petrosal n. to the                   ⎬ sensation, hyperacusis
lacrimal gland                       ⎭

Nerve to stapedius                   ⎫ Facial paralysis, loss of
                                     ⎬ taste sensation
                                     ⎭
Chorda tympani: taste fibres
to anterior two thirds of
tongue and motor fibres to           ⎫
the salivary glands                  ⎬ Facial paralysis
Stylomastoid foramen                 ⎭
Facial nerve
```

Fig. 26. The facial nerve and the disabilities caused by lesions at different sites along its course.

indicates when the sound disappears. The still ringing fork is then held in front of the ear, and the patient is again asked if he can hear the sound. If so, air conduction is better than bone conduction.

Weber's test. The base of a ringing fork is placed on the centre of the patient's forehead. He is asked whether the sound seems to come from the centre of his head or whether it is louder in one ear. The bone conducted sound reaches both cochleae with equal intensity, and thus normally seems to come from the centre of the head. Nerve deafness decreases the sensitivity on that side and so the sound appears to be louder in the healthy ear. Middle ear disease masks the extraneous air-conducted sound so that the sound conducted through the bone seems louder on the diseased side.

Audiometry. By this means the auditory threshold can be measured at different frequencies. The *recruitment test* enables the examiner to differentiate between deafness due to disease of the inner ear (e.g. Ménière's disease) and to nerve lesions. The intensity at which sound is first perceived is measured in both ears. The intensity is then increased in both ears by equal amounts. In recruiting (cochlear) deafness, the original discrepancy between the two ears eventually disappears, whereas in non-recruiting (nerve) deafness it persists.

Vestibular function
Spontaneous signs of vestibular disease are unsteadiness of gait and nystagmus. The patient tends to stagger towards the side of the lesion and this is exaggerated by closing his eyes.

Vestibular nystagmus. The fast phase is away from the side of the lesion. The lesion may be central (in the brain-stem) or peripherally placed and the site distinguished as follows. Peripheral vestibular nystagmus is usually in one direction only, it is short lasting (seconds) and the two eyes move conjugately. A central lesion causes long lasting or permanent nystagmus, which is multidirectional and the eyes move dysconjugately.

Tests of vestibular function
Caloric tests. Raising or lowering the temperature in the external auditory canal induces convection currents in the semicircular canals and stimulates the vestibular nerve endings.

The patient lies with his head raised by 30 degrees and his eyes fixed on a marked spot on the ceiling. Water at 44° C is run into the ear for 40 seconds. The duration of the nystagmus evoked is noted, and compared with the time for the other side. The test is repeated with water at 30° C. Nystagmus usually persists for 2–3·5 minutes. Disordered vestibular function is indicated by a diminished or absent response to caloric stimulation.

This test does not form part of the routine examination.

(IX, X) Glossopharyngeal and vagus nerves
The ninth and tenth nerves are closely related anatomically and are tested together.

The patient is asked to open his mouth and say 'ah'. The soft palate normally rises briskly and symmetrically. The ninth nerve carries common sensation from the posterior part of the tongue and the nasopharynx. Stimulation of the back of the throat with a spatula causes a gag reflex, the efferent pathway being by way of the vagus nerve.

The selective involvement of the recurrent laryngeal branch of the vagus can be recognized by examining the vocal cords with a laryngeal mirror. The cords are normally abducted during inspiration and adducted on coughing or speaking. With unilateral paralysis the affected cord lies in the mid-position and does not move. The healthy cord, however, moves over towards the affected side so that functionally the weakness is unrecognizable.

Taste sensation from the posterior third of the tongue is tested with the seventh nerve.

(XI) Spinal accessory nerve

(a) Branch to the sternomastoid. The patient is asked to turn his head to the opposite side and to resist the examiner's attempt to turn it back.

(b) Branch to the upper fibres of the trapezius. The patient is asked to shrug his shoulders against resistance.

(XII) Hypoglossal nerve

The patient is asked to protrude his tongue. This is normally done promptly and in the mid-line. Unilateral paralysis causes deviation of the tongue towards the affected side. If he puts his tongue in his cheek, the strength of this movement can be tested by the examiner. The tongue should be examined for evidence of lower neuron disease, namely atrophy and fasciculation.

Neck and trunk

The range of movement of the constituent parts of the spinal column should be tested. Any unusual pain, tenderness or rigidity, should be noted. Meningeal irritation causes a reflex retraction of the head and neck.

The trunk muscles are tested by asking the patient to raise himself from a supine posture, without the use of his hands. The paraspinal muscles are tested by asking him to raise his head and shoulders while lying prone. The respiratory excursion and movement of the diaphragm should be examined. All forms of sensation should be tested on the back and front of the trunk, including the perineal area.

The limbs

Power

There is no satisfactory quantitative method of measuring muscle strength. The examiner relies upon the patient's co-operation and a rough comparison with his own strength. The scale devised by the Medical Research Council is a convenient method of recording strength, but the use of numbers in itself does not make the assessment any more precise.

    0—no active contraction.
    1—visible or palpable contraction without active movement.
    2—movement with gravity eliminated.
    3—movement against gravity.
    4—movement against gravity plus resistance.
    5—normal power.

It is probably easier to develop a standardized technique if the muscles are tested when contracting isometrically. For example, when testing the biceps, the patient is told to bend his elbow and to resist the examiner's attempt to straighten his arm. Although this method may not reveal some of the lesser degrees of weakness, it has the advantage that the patient is in no doubt as to what is expected of him.

The routine examination should include an assessment of the following important movements:

Upper limbs:	Shoulder	Adduction, abduction, flexion and extension.
	Elbow	Flexion and extension.
	Wrist	Flexion and extension.
	Fingers	Flexion (grasp), extension, adduction, abduction and opposition of the thumb to the little finger.

Where indicated, a more detailed examination of the small muscles of the hand should be made.

Lower limbs:	Hip	Flexion extension, adduction and abduction.
	Knee	Flexion and extension.
Lower limbs:	Ankle	Dorsiflexion and plantar flexion, eversion and inversion of the foot.
	Great toe	Plantar flexion and dorsiflexion.

Tone

When the patient is accustomed to the examiner manipulating his limbs, an attempt may be made to assess the tone. This is made during the passive movement of joints through their normal range. Tone may be normal, decreased or increased. Spasticity is typified by maximal resistance at the beginning of the movement. Continued resistance throughout the range is called rigidity.

This is a convenient time to test the patient's **straight leg raising**. With the patient lying flat on his back the examiner raises each fully extended leg in turn. Normally the leg can be raised through 90 degrees. If the lumbar nerve roots are already under increased tension (e.g. from a prolapsed disc) the additional stretching causes painful reflex spasm. This prevents the full elevation of the leg.

Kernig's sign. With the knee bent, the thigh can be fully flexed against the abdomen. Attempts to straighten the knee meet resistance in cases of meningeal irritation or tension on the lumbosacral nerve roots.

Sensation

The sensory examination requires the co-operation and interest of the patient, and perseverance by the examiner. If there is doubt about the reliability of sensory findings it is better to repeat the test at a later date than to prolong the initial examination.

Touch, pain, temperature (hot and cold), vibration and muscle joint sense are tested. It should be determined whether sensation is normal, decreased, absent or heightened, and areas of abnormal sensation should be delineated. It is easier for a patient to recognize when sensation becomes more acute. Should an area of depressed sensation be found, then its boundaries can best be determined by first testing within this area and working out towards normal. In the routine examination only a sample of the body surface can be tested. The examiner should choose representative areas from each of the dermatomes of segmental innervation and from the distribution of the main peripheral nerves (Figs 6 and 7).

Light touch is tested using a piece of cotton wool. It should be a touch and not a tickle. Pain is tested with a pin. Temperature is tested using tubes containing hot and cold water. Muscle/joint sensation is tested by asking the patient to identify the direction of small movements at the distal interphalangeal joints. He is told to close his eyes. The examiner takes the middle phalanx firmly in his left hand, and with the index finger and thumb of his right hand grasps the sides of the terminal phalanx. The movements should be quite definite but of small amplitude. If sensation is absent distally then more proximal joints should be tested.

Vibration sense is tested with a 128 cycle per second tuning fork applied to the bony prominences.

Parietal lobe function tests include:

Stereognosis—the tactile recognition of shapes. With his eyes closed the patient is asked to:

1. Identify small objects which can be held in the hand, e.g. key, various coins, pocket knife.
2. Identify numbers written on the pulp of his finger.
3. Distinguish between single and dual stimuli applied close together (two-point discrimination).

Body schema. He is asked to identify parts of his body. This can be combined with tests of right/left orientation.

Sensory attention. His ability to recognize bilateral simultaneous stimuli is tested.

Praxis. He is asked to demonstrate how he would strike a match, use scissors and clean his teeth. He then should construct a simple geometric figure, such as a five-point star with matches.

Co-ordination. The ability to maintain a chosen posture and perform accurate voluntary movements is tested.

Postural maintenance. The patient is asked to hold out his arms in front of him.

Muscular weakness will make his arms droop whether his eyes are open or closed.

Disorders of joint position sense cause the arms to drift, more so when the eyes are closed.

Cerebellar disease. A sharp tap on the hand will cause exaggerated displacement, with excessive compensatory return and overshoot.

When the patient lies down, the legs can be tested in a similar way.

Normal upright stance demands a combination of these postural mechanisms with normal vestibular function. Sensory defects are exacerbated by asking the patient to close his eyes (Romberg's tests).

Co-ordinated voluntary movements. Finger/nose test. The patient is asked to touch his index finger on the tip of his nose. This will be performed clumsily if there is a motor or sensory deficit. Cerebellar disease results in fragmentation of the normally smooth continuous movement. The finger makes 'searching movements' which often become more pronounced near the target. This is called intention tremor.

Rapidly alternating movements—the patient should be asked to rotate his hands in the air, or tap rapidly with his fingers on the back of the examiner's hand. Cerebellar disease results in awkwardness, slowing and the employment of varying force in the performance of these movements. This is called dysdiadochokinesis.

Equivalent tests which are suitable for the examination of the legs are the heel/shin test and the heel tapping test.

Heel/shin test: The patient is told to run his heel down the front of his other leg.

Heel tapping test: He is asked to tap his heel rapidly on the front of his other leg.

Reflexes

The corneal reflex and the jaw jerk have already been described.

The tendon reflexes are elicited by applying a sudden stretch to the muscle which contracts reflexly through the monosynaptic spinal arc. The muscle stretch is produced by a sharp tap from a tendon hammer near the insertion of the tendon. The biceps, triceps, supinator (brachioradialis), knee and ankle jerks are tested.

Apart from deciding whether the reflexes are normal, increased or decreased, it is important to compare the reflexes from both sides of the body.

For eliciting the reflexes, the patient should be completely relaxed and the limbs arranged so that the muscles are stretched to about half their full range. In the upper limbs this position is approximated by asking the patient to sit with his hands held loosely in his lap.

Knowing the segmental innervation of any reflex may be helpful in determining the site of a lesion in the spinal cord or a nerve root (Table 1).

Sluggish lower limb reflexes may be augmented by asking the patient to hook the fingers of his two hands together and to try to pull them apart. Upper limb reflexes may be reinforced by asking the patient to clench his teeth.

In the presence of increased tone, *clonus* may be elicited at the knee and ankle. The ankle is sharply dorsiflexed and the pressure

Table 1. Segmental innervation of reflexes

Glabellar tap	Cn V (i) and Cn VII
Corneal	Cn V (i) and Cn VII
Jaw jerk	Cn V (iii) and Cn V
Biceps jerk	C 5—6
Supinator jerk	C 5—6
Triceps jerk	C 7—8
Abdominals Upper and Lower	T 9—12
Cremasteric	T 12—L 2
Knee jerk	L 3—4
Ankle jerk	S 1

on the foot is maintained. With the knee straight the patella is pushed downwards. True clonus should persist while the stretch is maintained.

A numerical code is convenient for recording the reflexes:

0 absent
1 diminished
2 normal
3 increased
4 clonus

Superficial reflexes are altered both by local segmental lesions and by disease of the upper motor neuron. The abdominal reflexes are elicited by stroking the skin of the abdominal wall. The four quadrants are tested and the strokes are drawn parallel to the margins of the rib cage and the groins from the flanks medially. A positive response causes a contraction of the muscles of the abdominal wall and displacement of the umbilicus. This reflex is commonly absent in the elderly and in multipara, and accompanying upper motor neuron disease. The cremasteric reflex is provoked by scratching the inner aspect of the thigh. The cremasteric muscle on the same side contracts and draws up the testicle.

The plantar reflex

The response is elicited by drawing a blunted object along the lateral border of the sole of the foot. In the absence of disease all the toes bunch together and plantarflex. The extensor plantar response is a sensitive indication of upper motor neuron disease. It consists of dorsiflexion of the great toe and fanning of the other toes. In a developing lesion the extensor response first appears to stimuli along the lateral border of the foot, later spreading medially.

Gait

The neurological examination is not complete without seeing the patient walk.
Some of the common disturbances of gait are:

1. *Hemispasticity:* The patient learns to walk with a twisting movement of the pelvis which lifts the spastic leg and swings it clear of the ground.

2. *Spastic paraparesis:* Small, shuffling steps.

3. *Cerebellar ataxia:* Staggering gait, wide-based, with the arms often flung out to maintain balance. This may be accompanied by titubation, a rhythmical shaking movement of the body and head.

4. *Sensory ataxia:* Wide-based, stamping gait, with eyes fixed on the ground. Falls when eyes are closed.

5. *Parkinsonism:* Posture stooped. The arms do not swing and are possibly flexed against the body. Small, shuffling steps, with a tendency to break into a tottering run. Slowness in initiating movements.

Mental state

A brief assessment of the patient's mental state should be part of every neurological examination. Some idea of the patient's awareness of his surroundings and his attitude towards his circumstances will become apparent while the history is taken. In addition, the examiner should record his

1. State of consciousness. Is he fully alert, drowsy, irritable, comatose?

2. Orientation. Does he know where he is, the date, the time of day?

3. Memory. Is his memory good for current events, recent history, and details of his past life? Can he retain a sequence of seven or eight digits?

4. Mood. Does he appear to be emotionally stable: is he depressed, excited, grandiose?

5. Intelligence. Are his reasoning powers and his understanding compatible with his type of employment and education?

6. Calculation. Can he make simple calculations, such as the 100–7 sequence?

Examination of the unconscious patient

The purpose of the examination is threefold: to identify the cause of unconsciousness; to locate any intracranial lesion; to recognize related systemic or metabolic disorders.

Eye-witness accounts of the illness should be sought so that its acuteness, and the occurrence of fits or injury may be determined.

A general examination should be made for signs of injury, especially injury to the head, evidence of infection, such as a raised temperature and neck stiffness; diabetic coma, uraemia or intoxication with alcohol or other drugs.

Raised intracranial pressure is recognized by papilloedema, a progressive bradycardia and arterial hypertension.

A recent fit may be suspected if the tongue or lips are bitten or if the patient has vomited or has been incontinent of urine. A more detailed examination is made for focal neurological signs. The symmetry of muscle tone, of spontaneous limb movements and the tendon reflexes are tested.

Static or progressive ocular signs are valuable indicators of brain-stem lesions.

1. Bilateral dilatation of the pupils is commonly related to the depth of unconsciousness.

2. Unilateral fixed dilated pupil suggests entrapment of the oculomotor nerve by herniation of the temporal lobe past the edge of the tentorium cerebelli.

3. Irregular non-reacting pupils: probably a mid-brain lesion.

4. Small non-reacting pupils: probably a pontine lesion.

5. Fixed lateral deviation of the eyes suggests a supranuclear lesion; perhaps in the cerebral hemisphere.

6. Dysconjugate eye movements are seen in brain-stem lesions.

Brain-stem reflexes. These responses depend upon normally functioning pontine/midbrain structures.

Doll's head manoeuvre; the patient's head is rotated laterally and vertically. The eyes normally move in the opposite direction to the movement of the head. Caloric responses (p. 72) are performed using ice-cold water.

Part III
Diseases of the Nervous System

Chapter 11
Epilepsy

Epilepsy comprises a group of conditions which are characterized by recurrent paroxysmal disorders of brain function.

The management of a patient who presents with episodes of altered consciousness requires:
1. An accurate clinical description of the attacks.
2. The differentiation of epilepsy from the other causes of altered consciousness.
3. The investigation of any pathological condition which may be responsible for the seizures.
4. Correction of the primary condition.
5. Symptomatic treatment.

DIAGNOSIS

While taking the history an attempt should be made to:
1. Get a complete description of the fit including any slight disturbance which may precede the convulsion.
2. Establish the patient's age at which the first attack occurred.
3. Determine the frequency of attacks and their relation to the time of day, other illnesses, emotional disturbances and, in the female, to the menstrual cycle.

A family history should include details of any neurological or mental illness and a note of any faints or fits. If the patient is a child his mother should be asked for details of the birth history. The possibility of birth injury is suggested by the use of instruments, prolonged or precipitate labour and an initial failure to thrive.

A previous history of head injury, encephalitis or meningitis may be significant.

The first clinical problem is the differentiation between epilepsy and those other conditions causing transient loss of consciousness. The most difficult is the distinction between syncope and epilepsy. Is it a fit or a faint? Drop attacks, hypoglycaemia, narcolepsy and hysterical manifestations are more easily recognized.

Syncope. A transient loss of consciousness due to cerebral ischaemia (p. 122). The onset is gradual and preceded by feelings of weakness, dizziness, nausea, hazy vision and sweating. The patient slips limply to the ground and seldom injures himself. He is pale and his pulse is of a small volume. If allowed to lie flat, recovery occurs after a minute or two and is usually gradual like the onset. Within a few minutes the subject feels quite normal. Incontinence of urine, tongue biting, headache, and postictal confusion are unusual.

Drop attacks. This term is used in two ways. Some authors describe a sudden fall to the ground with momentary loss of consciousness. This is a form of epilepsy. Others use the term for a sudden weakness of the legs making the patient fall—but without loss of consciousness. This is most commonly due to basilar artery insufficiency (p. 124) but a parasaggital meningioma or a third ventricle cyst may be responsible.

Hypoglycaemia. The onset of an attack is prolonged. It consists of sweating, light headedness, and sometimes a feeling of panic. There are periods of confusion and automatism. A time relationship to meals can sometimes be established. *Rebound hypoglycaemia* is due to an excessive output of insulin in response to a carbohydrate load. An insulin secreting adenoma or a therapeutic overdosage of insulin are other possible causes. Attacks can sometimes be provoked by a prolonged fast, or a tolbutamide test. The blood sugar in an attack is low, and intravenous glucose quickly restores the patient to normal.

Narcolepsy is manifest by irresistible diurnal attacks of sleepiness. In most cases it is an entirely benign condition, of unknown cause, first appearing in adolescence or early adulthood. Attacks occur most frequently when the patient is not physically active, for example while sitting in a bus or while reading. It has all the features of normal sleep: the onset is gradual, the eyelids begin to droop and the head nods. When falling asleep the patient may experience visual or auditory hallucinations *(hypnagogic hallucinations).* He wakens within a few minutes feeling perfectly fresh. Apart from the changes associated with normal sleep, the electroencephalogram is normal. Narcolepsy is usually alleviated by taking dexamphetamine sulphate 15 mg morning and mid-afternoon.

The same patient may also suffer from *cataplexy*. In this condition there is a sudden loss of muscle tone so that the subject crumples to the ground while remaining fully conscious. It is often precipitated by strong emotion such as laughter, anger or grief.

Hysterical fits. This expression of hysteria often coexists with epilepsy. A hysterical fit usually results in some apparent gain for the patient although he is seldom aware of his motivation. These attacks occur only in front of an audience. An attempt to examine the patient during an attack is met with active opposition and restraint causes increasingly violent convulsive movements. The patient may utter strange cries and the flailing limbs are a parody of a true epileptic convulsion. The plantar responses remain flexor and the pupils react to light throughout an attack.

Any attack which occurs during sleep should be regarded as epileptic. Except in the sophisticated hysteric, incontinence and tongue biting are indications of epilepsy.

Epilepsy is a symptom and not in itself a disease. It may be a symptom of:
1. Congenital neuronal dysfunction.
2. Systemic metabolic disorder.
3. Structural brain disease.

(1) Congenital neuronal dysfunction
The physiological stability of the neurons depends on the physical structure and chemical composition of their cytoplasmic membrane. Congenital predisposition to seizures is probably due to a chemical abnormality of the cell membrane. This allows sudden concerted neuronal discharges which give rise to the fit. The cause of this abnormality can seldom be determined. Thus it is known as idiopathic epilepsy (arising from itself), or cryptogenic epilepsy (of hidden origin). The site of this abnormally discharging focus is believed to be in the reticular formation of the upper brain stem, an area which Penfield called the centrencephalon. There is a spread of activity to the cerebral cortex and abnormal electrical discharges can be recorded with the electroencephalograph from all parts of the brain simultaneously. This is also called centren-

cephalic epilepsy. The disturbance in the brain-stem always causes loss of consciousness for a period, however brief.

(2) Systemic metabolic disorders
Circulating toxic substances or the deficiency of an essential nutrient may provoke discharges from the centres in the reticular formation giving rise to generalized convulsions.

Deficiencies
Hypoxia, hypoglycaemia, hypocalcaemia, pyridoxine deficiency.

Metabolic disorders
Uraemia, cholaemia; alterations in pH of the tissue fluids. Febrile illnesses in childhood are not uncommonly accompanied by convulsions; this may be due to the physical rise in temperature or to some endogenous toxin.

Exogenous toxic substances
Metrazol and other analeptics: lead.

The electroencephalogram may be normal but diffuse slow wave activity is often seen between attacks. During a fit the typical centrencephalic discharges occur.

(3) Structural brain disease
Almost any disease of the brain may give rise to a group of abnormally discharging neurons which form an epileptogenic focus. The nature of the ictus depends on the site of the responsible lesion (p. 90 *et seq.*), for example, a scar on the motor cortex might cause a focal motor seizure, with convulsive movements of the contralateral limbs. The fit may remain localized or there may be a spread of the discharge along the affected gyrus to involve other parts of the body (Fig. 27). There may be extension down to the reticular formation in which case a generalized convulsion will follow on the focal seizure. The electroencephalogram (EEG) usually provides evidence of the site of the epileptogenic focus.

Pathological tissue (e.g. tumour or abscess) is not itself epileptogenic, but oedema and other physical changes in the neurons on the edge of the lesion may form a discharging focus. Thus the localization of an intracranial lesion by means of the EEG is likely to be misleading unless this relationship is borne in mind. There may be a localized slow wave abnormality, or if the lesion is near the cortex, a 'spike' discharge is commonly seen.

Table 2. Relative frequency of cause of epilepsy related to age at first attack

	Age	Lesion
Infancy	0–2	Birth injury, degeneration, congenital abnormality
Childhood	2–10	Birth injury, febrile thrombosis, trauma, idiopathic
Adolescence	10–20	Idiopathic, trauma, birth injury
Youth	20–35	Trauma, neoplasm
Middle age	35–55	Neoplasm, trauma, arteriosclerosis
Senescence	55–70	Arteriosclerosis, neoplasm

From PENFIELD & JASPER (1954), *Epilepsy and the Functional Anatomy of the Human Brain*. Boston, Little Brown & Co.

Cerebral birth injury and developmental defects are the most common forms of gross brain disease associated with epilepsy. Cerebral tumour and abscess, and the degenerative disorders including vascular disease are the more common causes in later life. The age at which the first fit occurred determines the likeliest aetiology (Table 2).

In the foregoing discussion, two methods of categorizing epilepsy have been used. On the one hand these have been based on aetiology, and on the other hand on the clinical descriptions and the electroencephalogram. These methods are complementary (Table 3).

It is apparent that there must be several supplementary influences which will precipitate a fit. If a structural abnormality of the nerve cell membrane were the only factor then one might expect that the affected individual would have continuous seizures. Similarly, less than half of those who suffer penetrating brain injuries have fits, and thus the irritant focus is not the sole cause in these cases.

From a practical viewpoint, a consideration of these supplementary influences is worth while as they can sometimes be controlled or at least modified, and the frequency of attacks diminished. They include: fever, irregular and neglected meals, perhaps with attendant hypoglycaemia; over-hydration and water retention of menstrual origin; alkalosis and pH changes resulting from hyperventilation; lack of sleep; alcoholic excess; emotional disturbances and pregnancy.

Table 3. Complementary descriptions of epilepsy

Aetiological description		Clinical description	EEG
Idiopathic epilepsy	Principally due to congenital neuronal instability	Generalized fit (major and minor)	Centrencephalic epilepsy
Symptomatic epilepsy	Principally due to metabolic or toxic disorders		
	Principally due to structural brain disease	Focal attack	Focal epilepsy

CENTRENCEPHALIC EPILEPSY

Grand mal (major epilepsy)

If this type of fit develops in childhood or adolescence, it is likely to be the result of congenital predisposition. In later life it should be regarded as a symptom of progressive brain disease or metabolic disorder until it is proved otherwise.

During the days or hours before an attack the patient may experience feelings of irritability and various minor disturbances such as myoclonic jerks. The onset of the actual fit is sudden. There may be a momentary feeling of strangeness (the aura), but almost immediately the patient is struck unconscious and falls rigidly to the ground. This is the tonic phase characterized by powerful muscular contraction. Air is forced from the chest, sometimes in a loud cry, and the teeth are clenched. No respiratory movements occur and the patient becomes cyanosed. The tonic phase lasts for about half a minute and is followed by the clonic phase. This consists of violent convulsive movements of the limbs which occur at a gradually decreasing frequency. The lips, tongue or cheek may be bitten. The combination of relaxed sphincters and the contraction of the abdominal musculature may cause incontinence of urine and less often of faeces. The clonic phase is followed by a complete relaxation of the muscles, when the patient will sleep or rouse gradually. The period of unconsciousness generally lasts for a few minutes but may persist for several hours. All the tendon reflexes are depressed, the pupils are large and unreacting and the plantar reflexes are extensor. On recovering consciousness the patient is likely to be confused and may complain of headache, nausea and drowsiness.

In the inter-ictal period, the physical examination, the CSF and neuroradiography show no diagnostic abnormalities.

The electroencephalogram. On the rare occasions that an EEG is obtained during a fit, synchronous high voltage fast waves are recorded over all parts of the brain. Immediately after a fit, the record is often of low voltage and for the next few days it may contain focal slow wave activity which subsequently disappears. Between attacks, bilaterally synchronous wave and spike discharges or runs of symmetrical slow wave activity may be seen. A normal record does not preclude the diagnosis of epilepsy.

The frequency of attacks varies from two or three in a lifetime to several in one day. Large numbers occurring in succession are termed serial epilepsy. If consciousness is not regained between the attacks this is known as status epilepticus and its prolonged continuance threatens life.

Petit mal

This term has a very specific meaning but is much abused. The diagnosis should be made only when the first attacks occur during childhood and in the presence of the characteristic EEG pattern. It is always due to a congenital neuronal instability.

Petit mal consists of brief interruptions of consciousness, sometimes accompanied by rhythmical blinking of the eyelids. The child does not fall and frequently is unaware that anything has happened. To the lay observer he appears to be dazed or daydreaming. Recovery is immediate and there are no sequelae. Normally, petit mal attacks occur much more frequently than grand mal. Some patients may have several hundred attacks in one day. Such frequent attacks seriously interfere with education. Children with petit mal may also suffer major seizures. There is a tendency for petit mal to remit in adolescence.

Electroencephalogram. A 3 per second, spike and wave discharge synchronous in both hemispheres is characteristic of petit mal. This accompanies attacks and is often seen between the clinical attacks.

Special radiological investigations and the cerebrospinal fluid are normal.

Myoclonic epilepsy

A form of idiopathic epilepsy, developing in early childhood. Various types of generalized fits occur including sudden jerking movements of the limbs (myoclonus). The EEG shows the characteristic wave and spike pattern. Myoclonus is sometimes a symptom of serious structural disease of the brain.

FOCAL EPILEPSY

These attacks are symptomatic of previous or continuing structural brain disease. During a focal attack the patient remains conscious and this is sometimes described as minor epilepsy. Not uncommonly the discharge spreads to the brain-stem, causing loss of consciousness and a generalized convulsion.

The nature of the attack varies according to the primary site of the lesion (Fig. 27).

The pre-central motor cortex (focal motor attacks)
The seizure consists of clonic movements in localized groups of muscles, such as the hand or forearm. Rarely, such attacks may continue for hours or days in which case it is known as epilepsia partialis continuans.

The discharge may spread from its original focus, along the precentral gyrus causing a march of the clonic movements throughout the body. This is called a Jacksonian seizure. There are three common sites at which the seizure may develop: the corner of the mouth, the thumb and the great toe. Following a focal motor seizure there may be a short-lived weakness of that part of the body involved in the fit (Todd's paralysis).

The post-central sensory cortex (focal sensory attacks)
Either localized or spreading paraesthesiae occur. These are analogous to the motor attack originating in the pre-central cortex.

Epilepsy

The accessory motor cortex (adversive attacks)

Fits originating in this area begin with strong adversive movements of the head and eyes and less often involve the limbs. The head and eyes are turned towards the side opposite to the affected hemisphere and the contralateral arm may be raised at the shoulder. Sometimes the movements are highly organized and the patient walks in circles at the beginning of an attack.

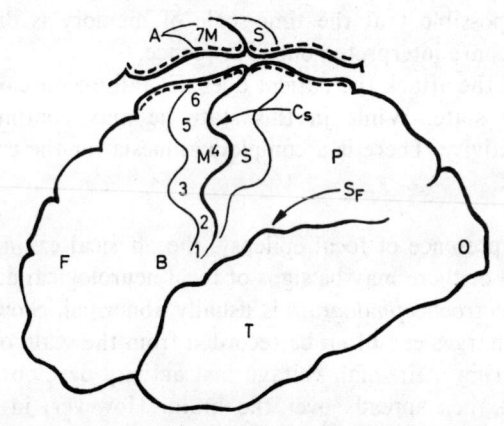

Fig. 27. Lateral view of the left cerebral hemisphere, with the adjacent part of the medial surface shown inset.
A. Accessory motor area. B. Broca's area. Cs. Central sulcus. F. Frontal lobe. M. Motor cortex. O. Occipital lobe. P. Parietal lobe. S. Sensory cortex. Sf. Sylvian fissure. T. Temporal lobe.

Representation of the body over the motor cortex: 1. Mouth. 2. Face. 3. Thumb. 4. Hand. 5. Arm. 6. Trunk. 7. Leg.

The temporal lobe

Temporal lobe seizures cause complex disorders of sensation. These consist of hallucinations of sight, sound, taste and smell, touch and memory. The hallucinations may be of simple sensory phenomena such as odours or single sounds, or may consist of highly developed psychic disturbances. The patient often has difficulty in identifying the sensory experience. The gustatory and olfactory hallucinations are usually rather unpleasant and may be accompanied by chewing movements and smacking of the lips. These are called uncinate fits. Hallucinatory voices and visions are not uncommon. The actual experience may be frightening or the patient may feel disquieted for no apparent reason. Less frequently it gives rise to a sense of ecstasy.

Two transient memory disturbances are characteristic of temporal lobe epilepsy: *jamais vu and déja vu*.

Jamais vu is a sudden feeling of unfamiliarity while the patient is in his own environment. *Déja vu* is a vivid sense of familiarity with the current situation. Although the experience may be quite new to the individual, he feels that 'it has all happened before'. It is difficult to explain the mechanism underlying these disorders but it seems possible that the time-scale of memory is disordered so that events are interpreted out of sequence.

During the attack the patient does not fall unconscious, but is in a dreamy state. While in this state he may continue with his normal activity. There is a complete amnesia for these events after the attack.

In the presence of focal epilepsy, the physical examination may be normal or there may be signs of focal neurological deficit.

The *electroencephalogram* is usually abnormal. Slow waves and spike discharges can often be recorded from the scalp overlying the focus. During a fit, high voltage fast activity develops first at the focus and then spreads over the brain. However, in the case of temporal lobe seizures, the slow wave discharge is commonly seen bilaterally.

Further investigation including skull X-rays, isotope scintiscanning, computer assisted tomography, and if necessary contrast radiography should be done in an attempt to identify and localize the lesion.

Epilepsy in childhood

In addition to petit mal, major convulsive seizures may occur.

In the newborn, cerebral birth injury, electrolyte disorders, hypocalcaemia, hypomagnesiaemia and hypoglycaemia may be responsible. Hypoglycaemia if untreated results in severe brain damage. It is more common in babies who are considered to be small for their calculated gestational dates, and whose mothers were ill during pregnancy. A blood glucose level of less than 1·5 mmol l^{-1} requires treatment by transfusion of i.v. glucose.

Of children who suffer from so-called infantile or febrile convulsions, about one-fifth will have fits in later life. Fits in childhood should be treated as each succeeding attack with its attendant cerebral anoxia gives rise to increasing neuronal damage.

Infantile spasms or salaam attacks occur in babies in the first year of life. They are characterized by sudden short-lived flexion of the trunk and interruption of consciousness. Commonly there is an associated retardation of mental development. The EEG shows recurrent high voltage complexes with progressive disruption of the intervening background activity (hypsarrhythmia). Conventional anticonvulsant therapy is ineffective. ACTH in doses up to 40 units daily controls the attacks, but does not reverse the mental slowing.

TREATMENT

Any primary structural or metabolic disorder should be corrected if this is possible. The symptomatic treatment of epilepsy then depends on the choice of appropriate drugs and help with establishing the patient in a suitable environment.

So far as is possible the patient should lead a normal active life. Under these circumstances he is likely to experience fewer seizures. Most children can attend an ordinary school, although the occurrence of frequent attacks may necessitate institutional care. Unnecessary exposure to heights, open machinery, fire and deep water should be avoided. Anyone subject to sudden alterations of consciousness is forbidden to drive. Children should not be allowed to go swimming unless supervised and parents should be reminded of the dangers for an epileptic child riding a bicycle. The frequency at which epilepsy occurs in the children of epileptics is not significantly greater than the frequency for the population in general, unless both husband and wife are epileptic. If advice is sought, such a match should be discouraged.

Drug treatment

The choice of drug and the dose depends on the type of fit, the patient's response and the occurrence of side effects. Individual responses to medication are variable. The ideal dose can be determined by measuring the serum levels of the drug. The most effective drug is chosen and if this is insufficient it can be supplemented with a second anticonvulsant. If two drugs are insufficient it is unlikely that the addition of further medication will be beneficial. Unwanted interactions may result from drug combinations.

Some drugs should be avoided as they potentiate an epileptic tendency. These include the phenothiazines and the barbiturates, with the exception of phenobarbitone.

Grand mal
Phenytoin is the drug of choice for adults. When used in childhood it often causes unsightly hirsutism, gum hypertrophy and thickening of the subcutaneous tissues. The therapeutic range is from 40–80 μmol l^{-1}. It is easily exceeded and careful dose adjustment is required.

Phenobarbitone (range 60–120 μmol l^{-1}) is a satisfactory treatment for adults although it may cause mental slowing. In childhood it worsens restlessness and behaviour disorders.

Primidone has a similar range of effectiveness and side effects to phenobarbitone. It is methylated to phenobarbitone in the body and the two drugs should not be given together.

Sodium valproate (range 350–700 μmol l^{-1}) is an effective treatment for centrencephalic epilepsy both grand mal and petit mal. Gastrointestinal side effects are common and weight increase is also a problem. It is suitable for adults and children.

Carbamazepine (17–34 μmol l^{-1}) is an excellent anticonvulsant, for adults and children.

Focal seizures
Phenytoin is the first choice in adults, and carbamazepine in children.

Petit mal
Sodium valproate is the drug of choice but ethosuximide (300–800 μmol l^{-1}) remains an effective alternative.

Anticonvulsants may activate or inhibit the effectiveness of other drugs by enzyme induction in the liver, e.g. the oral contraceptives. Osteomalacia may result from this complication.

Surgical treatment
This is only considered when a full trial with drug treatment has failed, when there is a clearly defined unilateral lesion and the underlying condition is static.

Treatment of a fit
The patient should be allowed to lie on the floor or bed without any attempt being made to restrain the convulsive movements. He should be removed from any place of danger, and a padded gag should be placed between his teeth. He should be turned semiprone.

Status epilepticus: repeated seizures without recovery of consciousness between attacks. This is a threat to life and demands urgent treatment.

Intravenous diazepam may be given as a single slow injection (10 mg) or in an infusion of saline or glucose (100 mg per 500 ml bottle). The rate of the drip is adjusted according to the patient's response.

Intravenous chlormethiazole or phenytoin are alternatives. Paraldehyde 10 ml IM still has a place in treatment and is without risk. In refractory cases curarization with controlled respiration may be necessary. The patient's routine anticonvulsant medication should be given throughout this period and when the fits are controlled close supervision is required until consciousness is regained. The usual measures for the care of an unconscious patient must be instituted (p. 100) with particular attention to the maintenance of the fluid and electrolyte balance.

Chapter 12
Cerebral Palsy

Cerebral palsy comprises a group of disorders of the motor system which are present at birth, although the first indication of disease may not be apparent until the child is more than a year old. There is much speculation regarding the cause of these disorders but, in general, there is an arrest in the development of selected neural systems during intrauterine life. This arrest is probably the result of a genetically determined defect in an enzyme system, or in the protein structure of the particular cell group. A number of preventable causes can be anticipated. Hypoxic cerebral damage antenatally may be due to placental insufficiency (fetal monitoring); postnatally it is often related to prematurity. Maternal infection with rubella or toxoplasmosis and Rh incompatibility can be identified.

The term cerebral palsy is sometimes broadened to include brain injuries and cerebral anoxia sustained during birth.

Perceptual (spatial) disorders are commonly associated with cerebral palsy. These increase the child's manipulative and educational difficulties and may give rise to an incorrectly low assessment of intelligence.

Spastic paraplegia
The clinical features are a spastic paraparesis with brisk tendon reflexes and extensor plantar responses which persist into the second year of life. Spasm of the adductor muscles of the thighs is usually prominent so that a scissors deformity is obvious if the child is lifted allowing the legs to hang free. The arms usually escape, but if they are involved (spastic quadriplegia) the spasticity and weakness is much less pronounced than that in the lower limbs. The abdominal reflexes are usually retained. Mental deficiency and epilepsy occur commonly.

The brain is small and sometimes the gyral development is immature. Microscopically the number of pyramidal cells in the motor cortex is diminished and myelination is incomplete.

Athetosis (p. 140)
The child with congenital athetosis is usually mentally normal, although the involuntary movements impair speech and make education difficult. The diagnosis often remains uncertain until the child begins to develop postural reflexes.

The neurons of the striatum are reduced in number and there is frequently a reactive gliosis.

Kernicterus (p. 140) may simulate congenital athetosis, but children with kernicterus are usually deaf and mentally defective.

Hemiplegia and double hemiplegia
The majority of children presenting with hemiplegia have a history of birth injury. In a quarter, the birth is quite normal and there is a unilateral agenesis of the brain. This is sometimes attributed to intrauterine cerebrovascular catastrophe.

The arm is more severely affected than the leg, and although the child may have seizures he is usually mentally normal. The condition may remain undiagnosed for several years until the patient presents with convulsions. A history of birth injury may be obtained, or asymmetry of the face and limbs may be detected.

Treatment
It is important to assess the child's intelligence, and then provide him with an appropriate education in a sheltered environment. Passive movements of the limbs are essential from an early age to prevent spastic contractures. At a later age, co-ordination exercises and speech therapy may be necessary. Anticonvulsants should be given to control seizures.

Chapter 13
Head Injury

Compound fractures and depressed fractures of the vault of the skull, and fractures through the base of the skull, require surgical treatment. Patients who sustain linear fractures should be observed for 24 hours, but in the absence of sequelae they require no special treatment.

BRAIN INJURY

There are three degrees of brain injury: concussion, contusion and laceration.

Concussion is a transient state of unconsciousness following head injury. It occurs without there being any gross damage to the brain. It may last for a few seconds or a few hours. If complete unconsciousness persists beyond this time then it is likely that more severe brain damage has occurred. After recovering consciousness the patient may be dazed and confused for 24 hours. Afterwards he remembers nothing of this period: this is called post traumatic amnesia. Loss of memory for events preceding the injury is known as retrograde amnesia. The duration of these states is an indication of the severity of the injury. Severe head injury causes alterations in the dynamics of the cerebrospinal fluid and the cerebral blood flow. Unconsciousness is probably due partly to mechanical distortion and partly to ischaemic changes in the reticular formation. Although there is no gross evidence of brain damage, experimental work has shown that concussion causes a widespread dissolution of nerve cells. Repeated concussion results in the 'punch drunk syndrome', consisting of intellectual impairment, mild tremor and rigidity.

Contusion and laceration are more severe forms of brain damage, with gross structural changes. Unconsciousness is prolonged. There is a danger of intracerebral haemorrhage and there is a likelihood of persistent neurological deficit after recovery. Deepening unconsciousness and signs of rising intracranial pressure (bradycardia, hypertension and a fall in the respiratory rate) may be due to haemorrhage or to cerebral oedema. Oedema may be lessened by the use of steroids (betamethasone) or by the slow intravenous infusion of hypertonic manitol (25 per cent).

Extradural haemorrhage
A fracture of the skull in the parieto-temporal region may tear the middle meningeal artery. As a result of this a haematoma develops in the extradural space. The sequence of events is diagnostic. The patient suffers a head injury and is unconscious for a short time. This is due to concussion. He recovers and is likely to feel quite normal. Some minutes or hours later he again sinks into coma. The increasing volume of blood within the extradural space raises the intracranial pressure, resulting in unconsciousness due to brain-stem compression.

Following a more severe head injury with cerebral contusion, an extradural haematoma may develop without the characteristic lucid interval.

An extradural haematoma requires immediate surgical attention.

Chronic subdural haemorrhage (haematoma)
Chronic subdural haematoma is a sequel to head injury in infants,

the debilitated and the elderly. The injury itself is often trivial and it may be weeks or months before it declares itself. The haemorrhage is due to the rupture of small veins crossing the subdural space. The blood becomes encysted and forms a serous pool between the dura and the arachnoid. Further expansion occurs by the absorption of fluid from the adjacent subarachnoid space. The onset of symptoms is characteristically insidious. Headache, mental changes, drowsiness and vomiting usually occur. There is often a mild hemiplegia but signs of raised intracranial pressure are not prominent. This causes herniation of the temporal lobes through the opening of the tentorium. Subsequent entrapment of the third nerve gives rise to ptosis and an enlarging pupil.

The initial symptoms and signs are easily attributable to cerebral arteriosclerosis. Early diagnosis depends upon the possibility being borne constantly in mind when fluctuating physical and mental changes occur in the elderly. Straight (AP) X-rays of the skull may show a displacement of a calcified pineal gland and, occasionally, calcification in the wall of the haematoma itself. Computerized axial tomography of the skull is likely to be diagnostic and is non-traumatic. The cerebrospinal fluid is under raised pressure and may be faintly yellow in colour. Contrast angiography shows that the vessels are pushed away from the vault of the skull.

All of these investigations may be negative, yet if the clinical state still suggests the presence of subdural haematoma, burr-holes should be made and the subdural space explored. No effort should be spared in the diagnosis, for the successful treatment of a haematoma results in a dramatic improvement in the patient's condition.

The post-concussional syndrome
This group of symptoms commonly follows head injury sustained at work. It is a rare sequel to sporting injuries and the relationship to unsettled claims for compensation has been stressed. It consists of headache, dizziness, fatigue, loss of confidence and depression. There are no objective physical abnormalities. Although the symptoms usually subside within a year or two, this condition may merge into a state of chronic psychoneurosis.

The syndrome can often be prevented if an enthusiastic and optimistic course of rehabilitation is instituted during the period of recovery from the original injury. Treatment of the established symptoms is seldom effective.

Post-traumatic epilepsy
Epilepsy may result from injury to the brain. The likelihood of this occurring is proportional to the severity of the injury.

The following factors are of value in predicting the eventual development of post-traumatic epilepsy:
1. A fit within a week of the injury.
2. Post-traumatic amnesia exceeding 24 hours.
3. Depressed fracture of the skull.
4. Intracerebral haematoma.

(Most cases of post-traumatic epilepsy are manifest within 2 years of the injury.)

The occurrence of two or more of the factors listed above are strong indications for recommending anticonvulsant therapy and the usual precautions against epilepsy for at least 2 years.

The unconscious patient

The survival of the unconscious patient depends on enthusiastic nursing care and constant medical supervision.

A chart should be kept to record changes in the level of consciousness, pulse rate, respiration, blood pressure, temperature and pupil size and reactions. The occurrence of vomiting and fits or any gross change in the neurological state should be noted. The frequency of observations will depend on the acuteness of the patient's illness and the stability of his clinical state. The examination of the unconscious patient is described on p. 80.

Routine care should be directed to the respiratory tract, the skin, the bladder and bowels, nutrition and control of the patient's temperature. Shearing damage to the hypothalamus may result in hyperpyrexia. Cooling with fans is usually sufficient to lower the temperature to normal. Chlorpromazine 25 mg–50 mg tds will lessen the tendency to shivering.

Sedatives should not be given. Any routine medication which the patient may have been receiving prior to the current illness should be continued—e.g. anticonvulsants and steroids.

Specialized investigations should include X-rays of the skull for signs of fracture and possible displacement of a calcified pineal gland. Computerized axial tomography for recognition of structural brain disease, haematoma, haemorrhage and oedema.

Angiography and echo encephalography are useful when CAT scanning is not available. Lumbar puncture may be hazardous and should be avoided unless infection is suspected.

Signs of brain death
An absence of all brain-stem reflexes.
Pupils fails to respond to bright light.
No corneal reflexes.
No vestibular responses to iced water irrigation.
No gag reflex.
No respiratory movements.

Chapter 14
Intracranial Tumour

The symptoms of an expanding intracranial lesion are caused by irritation and destruction of neural tissue and a rise in the intracranial pressure.

In the adult the cranium is a rigid bony box. The expanding intracranial lesion must displace or destroy the original contents. In childhood, before the skull sutures have fused, raised intracranial tension causes the sutures to spring apart. This can be recognized by the cracked pot note in response to skull percussion.

The site of a tumour and its rate of growth are the principal factors in determining the nature of its presentation. If the rate of growth is rapid, the surrounding structures are unable to accommodate the increasing bulk. This leads to distortion and displacement of the brain with the production of internal herniae. That is, the cerebral hemispheres are forced into the opening of the tentorium cerebelli, and the brain-stem and cerebellar tonsils are compressed in the foramen magnum. This in turn tends to obstruct the flow of cerebrospinal fluid, and exaggerates the increasing intracranial pressure. The symptoms attributable to *raised intracranial pressure* are headache, vomiting and dulling of consciousness. The pulse and respiratory rates are slowed, the blood pressure rises, and examination of the optic fundi reveals papilloedema. The development and progression of such signs is an indication for urgent surgical treatment.

Rapidly growing tumours are usually malignant and invasive. Destruction of cerebral tissue and the consequent functional deficit are characteristic features. The symptoms of a slowly expanding tumour often develop insidiously. The surrounding areas of the brain are compressed, but loss of function is a relatively late feature. Irritative phenonema such as focal seizures are much more common (p. 90). Papilloedema and the symptoms of raised intracranial pressure occur late unless the tumour is so sited that it obstructs the flow of cerebrospinal fluid.

These general principles governing the development of signs and symptoms apply to intracranial abscess and haematoma as well as to intracranial tumour. The differentiation of these space-occupying lesions is eminently worthwhile. In certain instances the appropriate treatment can result in a complete recovery.

The progressive development of physical signs is a most significant factor in the diagnosis of cerebral tumour.

From knowledge of its site, its clinical presentation and the age of the patient, one can make a fairly accurate diagnosis of the type of tumour. This assessment is aided by special investigations such as X-ray of the skull, computerized axial tomography, electroencephalography, brain scan, pneumo-encephalography and angiography. The final diagnosis, however, remains uncertain until a histological examination has been done.

Brain tumours are classified as primary, if arising *de novo* in the intracranial tissues, or secondary if their origin is in some extracranial organ such as the lung or breast. The majority of primary brain tumours are derived from glia, the meninges, the Schwann cells of the cranial nerves, the pituitary gland and from embryological cell rests.

Intrinsic brain tumours

This title embraces all tumours arising from the primitive neuro-ectoderm. The great majority are gliomas, i.e. tumours derived from the glial cells. The commonest is the astrocytoma, and such tumours are often graded from one to four according to their degree of histological differentiation. Grade I includes those tumours composed of highly differentiated cells which most nearly resemble normal astroglia. They are relatively benign and slow growing. Grade IV includes the most malignant tumours composed of poorly differentiated cells. These are reminiscent of the embryological blast cells from which glial tissue develops. The grade IV astrocytoma is commonly called a glioblastoma referring to this primitive cell structure. A grade I astrocytoma may after many years change to a less well-differentiated form, and a single tumour may be composed of cells which are of various grades of differentiation.

In adults, the astrocytoma is found most commonly in the cerebral hemispheres. A glioblastoma enlarges rapidly destroying the normal brain tissue in its path. It is highly invasive and its boundaries being difficult to determine make it unsuitable for surgical removal. The tumour is supplied by a tangle of fine blood vessels. Haemorrhage from these abnormal vessels into a necrotic area of the tumour causes sudden changes in the patient's clinical state. Headache, failure of memory, drowsiness, convulsions and progressive functional loss, developing over a period of a few weeks, characterize the malignant astrocytoma. The grade I astrocytoma is a slow growing tumour which is often cystic. It is relatively amenable to surgical treatment yet recurrence is almost inevitable. This is due to the difficulty entailed in removing the strands of tumour tissue which infiltrate the adjacent parts of the brain.

Both generalized and focal seizures precede the development of raised intracranial pressure by months or years. The site of the tumour can be established according to the principles discussed in Chapter 5.

The other types of glioma are the ependymoma and the oligodendroglioma. The ependymoma is fairly common. It grows from the ventricular wall into the cavity of the ventricle, tending to obstruct the flow of CSF. It also invades the adjacent brain tissue. The oligodendroglioma is uncommon.

The posterior fossa is the most common site for brain tumours in childhood. A relatively benign form of astrocytoma occurs in the cerebellar hemispheres, giving rise to ataxic voluntary movements and nystagmus. The results of surgical treatment are good.

The other common posterior fossa tumours in childhood are ependymomas growing into the fourth ventricle and the medulloblastoma. This is not a glioma, as the tumour cells retain the potential of maturing into cells of the neuronal series. It is a rapidly growing, soft and often necrotic tumour. It most commonly originates in the cerebellar vermis. An ataxic gait and poor postural control are prominent features. Papilloedema is found in almost every case. The medulloblastoma is sensitive to radiotherapy and this is usually combined with a subtotal resection. The tendency for this tumour to seed throughout the subarachnoid space makes it necessary to irradiate the whole length of the spine.

Meningioma

The meningioma is a firm rounded tumour composed of whorls of arachnoidal cells. It arises from the meninges close to the arachnoid granulations and thus the majority are found near the venous sinuses. Growing from the falx, the meninges of the base of the skull, or adjacent to the Sylvian fissure, it projects into, but does not invade, the brain. It has a rich blood supply derived from the meninges and hence the external carotid circulation. The richness of the blood supply accounts for some of the difficulties encountered in removing this benign tumour. The overlying skull is also highly vascularized. In about 25 per cent of cases, strands of tumour tissue penetrate the bone. These become ossified giving rise to short bony spicules raised from the inner and outer surfaces of the skull (hyperostosis). Meningiomas of the olfactory groove and the lesser wing of the sphenoid are attended by characteristic signs.

Olfactory groove meningioma: Unilateral anosmia and optic atrophy and euphoria. With enlargement of the tumour, bilateral anosmia and contralateral papilloedema develop.

Sphenoidal ridge meningioma: Protopsis, optic atrophy and involvement of the nerves to the extraocular muscles causing ptosis and diplopia. A superficial prominence of the temple is sometimes seen.

Acoustic nerve tumour

This tumour arises from the Schwann cells of the eighth cranial nerve. Like the meningioma, which it may resemble clinically, it compresses but does not invade the brain. A similar tumour is uncommonly seen in relation to the trigeminal nerve. Sometimes an acoustic nerve tumour is part of a generalized neurofibromatosis (von Recklinghausen's disease). It originates in or near the internal auditory meatus. If an acoustic nerve has given rise to clinical signs, then X-rays of the skull will almost invariably show erosion of the meatus. There will be symptoms of both auditory and vestibular dysfunction, and later the seventh and fifth nerves are involved. As the tumour expands in the angle between the pons and cerebellum, both of these structures will be compressed. The surgical removal of this tumour is attended by considerable technical difficulty.

Pituitary tumour

The most common tumour of the pituitary gland is a chromophobe adenoma. It expands within the pituitary fossa resulting in the destruction of the functioning gland. Symptoms of hypopituitarism develop insidiously and may be neglected for several years. Decreased libido, a reduction of body hair, and amenorrhoea; an increase in weight and intolerance of cold are commonly found. As the tumour enlarges the pituitary fossa is ballooned. Expansion beyond the confines of the fossa compresses the optic chiasm eventually giving rise to a bitemporal hemianopia. At first the patient may be unaware of his diminishing visual fields and complains only of headache and blurring of central vision.

The tumour can be delineated by computerized axial tomography. The treatment of choice is surgical, particularly if vision is threatened. Excision of the tumour is supplemented by steroid replacement therapy. Further deterioration of vision is prevented in all cases, and in about three-quarters there is improvement within a few weeks.

Less commonly, an eosinophil adenoma of the pituitary occurs. This causes hyperpituitarism resulting in gigantism in children and acromegaly in adults. In acromegaly there is overgrowth of the bones of the skull, the jaw, the hands and feet, and thickening of the skin and subcutaneous tissues of the face, tongue and hands. The tumour enlarges within the pituitary fossa, causing headache, but seldom compresses the optic chiasm. This tumour is usually treated with radiotherapy.

Craniopharyngioma

This suprasellar tumour, which also causes bitemporal hemianopia, occurs most frequently in childhood. It develops from embryological cell rests of Rathke's pouch. It is frequently cystic and contains areas of calcification which are visible on straight X-rays of the skull. It compresses both the hypothalamus and the pituitary gland causing delay in the development of secondary sexual characteristics, and abnormal deposition of body fat. The child complains of headache and poor vision. Examination reveals bitemporal hemianopia and, frequently, papilloedema. Complete surgical resection is often impossible due to the site of the tumour and involvement of adjacent vital structures.

Secondary tumours

Carcinoma of the lung, breast and bowel commonly metastasize to the brain. The deposits are frequently multiple and their clinical presentation is like that of a malignant astrocytoma.

THE INVESTIGATION OF INTRACRANIAL TUMOURS

Special investigations only supplement a carefully taken history and examination. This must include a general examination and a routine straight X-ray of the chest. In many instances, further investigation is not required for diagnostic purposes, but to provide the surgeon with a precise anatomical localization.

The investigations which are least likely to be traumatic should be chosen in preference to those with a recognized morbidity.

Plain X-ray films
Lateral, antero-posterior and Towne's views of the skull should be taken. These should be examined for:
  1. Signs of raised intracranial pressure. Spreading of the sutures and the beaten silver appearance in childhood. Decalcification of the clinoids in adults.
  2. Shift of the pineal gland. A calcified pineal gland marks the mid-line in the antero-posterior views.

Intracranial Tumour

3. Erosion of the skull over malignant tumours. Erosion of the internal auditory meatus. Ballooning of the pituitary fossa.
4. Hyperostosis, related to meningiomas.
5. Pathological calcification.

Electroencephalography
Tumour tissue is electrically silent. Disturbances of metabolism in the brain cells on the fringe of a tumour give rise to abnormal slow wave activity.

Computerized axial tomography of the skull: a technique producing enhanced radiological definition of the normal intracranial structures and an accurate demonstration of space occupying lesions. When available, this method of investigation has lessened the necessity for some of the invasive techniques.

Radioactive brain scanning
Highly vascular lesions show an increased uptake of various radio isotopes. Radioactive sodium pertechnetate ($NaTc^{99} NO_4$) is now used extensively. Potassium perchlorate or potassium iodide is given as a blocking dose to prevent excessive radiation to the thyroid. AP and lateral brain scans are then made. Meningiomas are well demarcated: astrocytomas and secondary tumours have a lower differential uptake ratio.

Angiography
This may show a displacement of the normal vascular pattern or reveal abnormal vessels.

Pneumoencephalography
This is a radiological technique for displaying the ventricular system using air as a contrast medium. Lumbar pneumoencephalography is of particular value for the definition of the basal cisterns and lesions in the posterior fossa. Like lumbar puncture, it is contraindicated in the presence of papilloedema. In this case, air may be injected directly into the ventricular system (ventriculography). It entails a minor surgical operation in which a burr hole is made in the skull, so that a cannula can be introduced directly into the lateral ventricle. By using myodil as the contrast medium a more precise demonstration of the aqueduct and fourth ventricle is sometimes obtained.

Chapter 15
Infections of the Nervous System

BRAIN ABSCESS

A compound fracture of the skull is a potential source of intracranial infection. Brain abscesses are otherwise secondary to suppurative disease elsewhere in the body. They may be due to a direct spread of infection from structures adjacent to the brain, or result from a blood-borne metastasis of septic material. The majority are secondary to chronic suppurative otitis media, and thus the most common site for a brain abscess is in the temporal lobe or the cerebellar hemisphere. The spreading infection occasionally gives rise to an extradural or subdural abscess. These are uncommon and the rarity of meningitis complicating an abscess suggests that the route of infection is probably along thrombosed veins (septic thrombophlebitis). This is also the source of intracranial infection secondary to cellulitis of the face.

The ready availability of antibiotics has reduced the incidence of chronic infection, with the result that bronchiectasis and lung abscess are now relatively uncommon sources of metastatic infection. Disease of the heart may be indirectly responsible. The presence of a septal defect allows septic emboli to bypass the normal filtering mechanism of the lung (paradoxical embolism). The septic emboli of bacterial endocarditis may give rise to a cerebral abscess which develops subsequent to a stroke.

The lodgement of septic material in the brain first causes a localized encephalitis. The surrounding tissue becomes inflamed, oedematous and softened. During this phase of the illness, the symptoms are attributable to the systemic effects of infection. Malaise, anorexia, headache and fever dominate while the symptoms of local brain damage may be insignificant. Vigorous treatment at this stage with sulphonamides and penicillin can prevent the establishment of an abscess.

The second phase in the development is for the centre of the infected area to undergo necrosis. This forms the abscess cavity which fills with pus. It eventually becomes walled off by a layer of granulation tissue surrounded by a reactive gliosis. At this stage,

Infections of the Nervous System

the symptoms are those of a space-occupying lesion. Both focal symptoms and more generalized symptoms due to raised intracranial pressure are found (p. 102). The more common site in the temporal lobe causes congruous field defects with speech disturbances if the abscess is in the dominant hemisphere. Temporal lobe seizures may occur. A cerebellar abscess gives rise to ipsilateral ataxia, muscular hypotonia and nystagmus.

An abscess may occasionally rupture into the ventricles or subarachnoid space causing a meningitis, but more often there is a non-specific meningeal reaction, with a slight increase in the protein of the CSF and 50–100 lymphocytes per mm^3. The sugar and chloride content are normal and no organisms are seen. There remains a high mortality in spite of treatment.

Diagnosis

A cerebral abscess should be suspected in any individual who, suffering from chronic sepsis, develops the signs of intracranial disease. In addition to the symptoms of systemic infection, headache, vomiting, drowsiness and generalized convulsions occur. The margins of the optic discs are often blurred, but gross papilloedema is uncommon. The appropriate investigations are those indicated in the section on cerebral tumour (p. 106).

Treatment

Treatment is aimed at suppressing the local infection, and sterilizing the contents of the abscess. This is achieved by giving the patient large doses of sulphadiazine, 4 g initially and then 1 g every 4 hours, and penicillin 3 million units six-hourly. Treatment is undertaken in close consultation with the neurosurgeons. Unless there is an immediate threat from raised intracranial pressure, the decision to drain the abscess is usually delayed until signs of local infection have been suppressed.

Having localized the abscess by appropriate radiological techniques, burr-holes are made, and the contents of the cavity are aspirated. Antibiotics are given systemically during this procedure. In some centres, antibiotics are also introduced directly into the abscess cavity, together with a radio-opaque dye such as Steripaque. X-rays of the skull are then taken on each subsequent day to demonstrate any changes in this size of the abscess. Further aspirations may be necessary. The final decision to remove the wall of the abscess is dictated by the circumstances of the individual case. This irritant focus is potentially epileptogenic and the patient should be given an anticonvulsant such as phenobarbitone 30 mg three times a day.

Treatment is not complete until the source of the infection has been defined and eradicated.

BACTERIAL MENINGITIS

Meningitis is an inflammation of the membranous coverings of the brain and spinal cord. Such inflammation may be due to infection or the introduction of an irritant sterile substance into the subarachnoid space, for example, subarachnoid haemorrhage or air during encephalography. Infection may be blood-borne or due to direct spread from an adjacent focus of infection.

The outstanding features of meningitis are headache, neck stiffness and clouding of consciousness. The diagnosis is confirmed by examination of the cerebrospinal fluid. The accumulation of a purulent exudate over the base of the brain sometimes affects the emerging cranial nerves, particularly giving rise to ocular palsies.

Acute purulent meningitis

Primary purulent meningitis in adults is almost always due to infection with the meningococcus. *Haemophilus influenzae* and *E. coli* are sometimes responsible for infection in childhood. Although sporadic cases do occur, meningococcal meningitis is primarily an epidemic disorder appearing when young people are crowded together. The disease is spread by droplet infection, and the organism lodges and multiples in the nasopharynx. It enters the bloodstream giving rise to a generalized septicaemia, pyrexia and malaise. Invasion of the meninges causes rapidly worsening headache, neck stiffness and deepening drowsiness. There are signs of cerebral irritability. Photophobia, increased tendon reflexes, vomiting and generalized or focal convulsions may occur. A haemorrhagic rash is sometimes seen.

The cerebrospinal fluid is under increased pressure and is cloudy or purulent. There are innumerable polymorphonuclear leucocytes and a smear stained with Gram's stain may demonstrate the organism. The CSF protein is greatly increased, the glucose is much reduced or absent, and the chlorides are also reduced.

The isolation of pneumococcus, staphylococcus or streptococcus from purulent cerebrospinal fluid is indicative of a secondary invasion of the meninges; this may be from an adjacent infected site or the result of a bacteraemia. The diagnosis is not complete until the primary site has been uncovered. Sepsis in the middle ear or sinuses and fracture through the base of the skull are frequent causes.

Clinically, these infections may be indistinguishable from meningococcal meningitis although the patient is often more seriously ill and his response to treatment is less predictable.

A dense purulent exudate forms over the base of the brain and extends towards the convexity along the sulci. In secondary meningitis it tends to be more profuse. Sulcal pockets of the exudate may become encysted or it may occlude the foramina of Magendie and Luschka with consequent hydrocephalus.

Treatment

Meningococcal meningitis. Treatment should be started immediately. As resistance to sulphonamides is increasing the first choice is benzyl penicillin. In adults 1·2–1·8 g i.v. four-hourly. Should the organism prove to be sensitive to sulphonamides, sulphadiazine 1 g four-hourly should be given. Treatment should be continued for three days after the patient is free from symptoms, a minimum total of eight days. If the patient is a child and there is any doubt about the causative organism, it is advisable to add chloramphenicol to the immediate drug schedule. When bacteriological confirmation of meningococcus is obtained the chloramphenicol may be discontinued.

Secondary meningitis. Treatment should begin with penicillin, 3 mega units six-hourly, supplemented with sulphadiazine in the dosage suggested for meningococcal meningitis. Additional intrathecal penicillin should be given to any patient who is seriously ill. The maximum single dose for an adult is 15 000 units of crystalline penicillin, dissolved in 10 ml of normal saline. This is given twice in the first 24 hours and then once daily until symptomatic improvement occurs. If the organism proves to be resistant to penicillin then the choice of antibiotic is dictated by its bacteriological sensitivity. There is a likelihood of relapse and antibiotic therapy should be continued for 10 days after the patient has made a clinical recovery.

Tuberculous meningitis

Tuberculous meningitis is a secondary manifestation of tuberculosis elsewhere in the body. The primary lesion may have gone unrecognized, but the most common site is in the lungs. Tuberculous meningitis is usually part of a miliary spread of infection. Less often it results from the discharge of a caseating tuberculoma in the brain. The meninges over the base of the brain are most severely affected. Here a tough gelatinous exudate often involves the cranial nerves and the blood vessels. The subsequent arteritis may lead to occlusion of the vessel and infarction of the tissues which it supplies. In the case of miliary dissemination, choroidal tubercles can often be found in the optic fundi. They are raised whitish-yellow spots about a quarter of the size of the optic disc.

It is primarily a disease of young people. The early symptoms are non-specific, consisting of malaise, loss of appetite, headache and a variable mild pyrexia. These symptoms may persist for a few days or a week or two. A gradual but unremitting deterioration occurs. The patient's headache becomes severe and changes of personality are sometimes noticed. Although there may be intermittent dulling of consciousness, periods of lucidity even in the most serious phases of the illness are characteristic. Vomiting, photophobia, convulsions and generalized irritability occur but are less prominent than in purulent meningitis. Mild neck stiffness and variably extensor plantar reflexes are found on examination.

Lumbar puncture reveals clear fluid under increased pressure. If allowed to stand, the fluid may form a faint web, but this also occurs in benign lymphocytic meningitis and other conditions where there is a moderate increase in the CSF protein. The protein is raised from $0.5-1.0$ g/l: up to 200 lymphocytes per cu mm are seen; the sugar falls to below 1.5 mmol/l, and the chloride below 118 mmol/l. Bacteriological confirmation is often delayed until the result of guinea-pig inoculation is available.

Treatment

The best chance of recovery is ensured by early vigorous treatment. Systemic treatment with isoniazid and rifampicin should be started. Isoniazid crosses the blood/brain barrier freely to enter the cerebrospinal fluid. 10 mg/kg daily are given in two divided doses. In the severely ill patient, isoniazid may be given intrathecally. The daily dose is 25 mg in 5 ml of normal saline. This should be given for one week or until clinical improvement occurs. Rifampicin is given in a dose of 600 mg daily. Streptomycin, 1 g daily, plus ethambutol, 25 mg/kg per day, are given for the first 3 months of treatment. Pyridoxine, 40 mg daily, is given to prevent the neurotoxic effects of isoniazid. When the lumbar puncture is performed, the pressure should be measured. If it is in excess of 200 mm, 10 ml of CSF should be drained. This helps to relieve the headache.

Children under one year of age should be given 5–10 mg of prednisolone daily to minimize formation of adhesions at the base of the brain. Phenobarbitone, 30 mg twice daily, is given as an anticonvulsant.

Systemic medication should be continued for at least one year. This is also governed by the patient's general state and the response of the primary lesion. The effect of treatment on the meningitis is assessed by the CSF glucose levels and the cell count.

NEUROSYPHILIS

Although neurological symptoms may not appear for fifteen or twenty years after the primary infection, more than half of the cases of neurosyphilis develop in the first three years. The blood-borne spirochaete *(Treponema pallidum)* may give rise to a mild *meningitis* within a few months of the initial infection. This uncommon presentation consists of severe and persistent headache with slight neck stiffness. Otherwise the patient appears to be quite well. Lumbar puncture produces clear fluid under increased pressure. There is a high lymphocyte count (200–500 cells per mm^3) and the protein is raised. The Wasserman reaction (WR) which is almost always positive differentiates this condition from acute lymphocytic meningitis of viral origin.

Meningovascular syphilis

Meningovascular syphilis occurs within five years of the primary infection. It consists of a low grade inflammatory process involving the arteries and the meninges. The nervous tissue is only secondarily involved.

Arteritis. All coats of the artery are affected, and the resulting fibrous proliferation narrows and sometimes occludes the vessel. This is known as endarteritis obliterans. It causes ischaemia or infarction in that part of the brain or spinal cord supplied by the affected artery. Cerebral ischaemia due to endarteritis is indistinguishable from that due to atherosclerosis. Endarteritis of the spinal arteries causes a meningomyelitis, with the signs of an incomplete transverse cord lesion, e.g. spastic paraparesis and diminished posterior column sensation (p. 54).

An exudative **meningitis** over the base of the brain commonly involves the third, fourth and sixth cranial nerves, giving rise to ptosis and diplopia. Proliferative meningitis in the cervical region results in compression of the emerging anterior and posterior nerve roots. This causes pain and numbness if the posterior roots are most affected, and a lower motor neuron lesion if the anterior roots are involved. The resultant wasting and fasciculation of the small muscles of the hands is called *syphilitic amyotrophy*. It may mimic motor neuron disease.

Parenchymatous neurosyphilis

In tabes dorsalis and general paralysis of the insane, the infection primarily affects the neural tissue. Only in general paresis has the spirochaete actually been identified in the nerve cells. Both forms are uncommon and occur more often in men than in women. The primary infection frequently goes unrecognized but is likely to have occurred about ten years before the development of neurological symptoms.

Tabes dorsalis

This name refers to the flattening of the dorsal columns seen when the spinal cord is examined.

There is a mild meningeal reaction but the site of maximum damage is in the posterior nerve roots. Although the pathogenesis has not been defined, it is assumed that the spirochaetes invade the posterior root ganglia. This results in the destruction of the nerve cell bodies and proximal degeneration of the fibres in the posterior nerve roots. The degeneration extends as far as the first synapse. In distinction from the other nerve fibres, those subserving muscle joint sensation enter the ascending tracts without first synapsing in the posterior horns. Thus, the posterior (dorsal) columns also

Infections of the Nervous System

undergo degeneration to give the characteristic pathological appearance. The lumbar nerve roots are most severely affected and lower limb symptoms predominate.

The symptoms may be interpreted in the light of the lesions in the posterior root ganglia and the cranial nerves.

Pain, numbness, ataxia, trophic changes, and diminished reflexes are the result of posterior nerve root lesions.

Pain. This is the earliest symptom, which sometimes starts as an intermittent dull ache. This may seem to originate from a joint so that the patient complains of rheumatism or arthritis. It soon develops the more usual searing, stabbing qualities, either penetrating deep in the tissues or running superficially along the course of the peripheral nerves. These are called lightning pains. Burning, constricting sensations may encircle the trunk. Acute abdominal pain associated with vomiting, the so-called visceral crisis, is an uncommon event.

Numbness. All forms of sensation may be lost in the affected segments. Superficial pain sensation is diminished and the areas of maximal anaesthesia are curiously localized to the medial border of the arms, the shins, the area round the nose, and the lower thorax. When testing pain sensibility, there is often a striking delay before the patient appreciates the pin prick.

Joint position sense is lost early causing *ataxia* which is most pronounced when the patient closes his eyes. He feels the ground soft or sandy under his feet and walks with a stamping gait. The tendon reflexes are lost.

Painless arthropathies may develop due to a blunting of deep pain sensation. Repeated minor injuries to the joint go unnoticed until severe damage with erosion and dislocation of the weight bearing surfaces has occurred (Charcot's joint). Similar painless joint deformities are found in syringomyelia. Trivial injuries to the soles of the feet are often ignored with the eventual development of penetrating ulcers.

Lesions in the sacral roots interrupt the afferent pathways from the bladder. Bladder sensation and the normal voiding reflexes are lost. The patient develops an atonic bladder, with retention and overflow incontinence (p. 27).

Primary optic atrophy occurs, but is uncommon. The patient complains of blurred vision and there is a concentric diminution in the visual fields. The optic disc is white and its margins are sharply defined.

Nerve deafness may also occur.

Argyll Robertson pupils are a characteristic finding in tabes. The pupils are small and irregular in shape. They react to convergence but not to light (p. 35).

The WR is positive in the blood and cerebrospinal fluid in 75 per cent of cases.

General paralysis of the insane (general paresis: GPI)

It is thought that the spirochaete gains access to the brain within a year or two of the primary infection. The route of entry from the blood stream is probably through the choroid plexus into the ventricular cerebrospinal fluid. The organism penetrates the cerebral tissue causing destruction of the cortical cells. There is a subsequent gliosis and shrinking of the brain.

The ventricles are enlarged and the sulci widened, especially over the anterior two-thirds of the brain.

The earliest symptoms are of **mental disorder.** This is at first slight and confined to an impairment of memory and difficulty in concentration. It soon becomes apparent that more serious mental changes are occurring, and the patient shows signs of a progressive dementia. Its nature varies from individual to individual: most are apathetic, some agitated, some depressed and some hallucinated. Self-aggrandizement may occur, but is not common. The patient usually complains of a diffuse but persistent headache. His speech is thick and slurred, some of the slurring being due to a tremor of the lips and tongue. There is also a tremor of the outstretched arms. The basal ganglia are sometimes more prominently involved giving rise to a form of parkinsonism.

The structure of the motor cortex is seriously disorganized and there is a consequent **spastic weakness** of the limbs with brisk reflexes and extensor plantar responses. Convulsions occur in about half of the cases. Most of these are generalized, but in some instances they are the result of localized cerebral haemorrhage or arteriolar thrombosis. The resulting paralysis is usually slight.

Diagnosis

The Wasserman reaction (WR) is positive in only about 50 per cent of cases. The fluorescent treponemal antibody test (absorbed) is specific for syphilis and remains positive in spite of successful treatment. The activity of the infection is gauged by the protein and cellular content of the CSF.

Cerebrospinal fluid

In all forms of active neurosyphilis there is an increase in the number of lymphocytes and the protein content. Lymphocytes number from 25–200 per mm^3, usually at the higher end of the range in meningovascular syphilis. The protein is raised from 0·5–1·2 g/l. The actual figures are of little help in distinguishing between the different forms. The colloidal gold curve differentiates general paresis (first zone) from tabes (mid-zone). The effect of treatment is first seen as a fall in the lymphocyte count. The protein and the gold curve remain elevated for several months after a curative course of treatment. The WR may remain abnormal for up to five years.

Treatment

Procaine penicillin 1·2 million units a day for 12 days is the treatment of choice for all forms of neurosyphilis. The cerebrospinal fluid should be re-examined three months after the course of treatment. If there has not been an appreciable fall in the cell count or if there has been any clinical deterioration, a further 15-day course of penicillin should be given.

Six months after an effective course of treatment, the cell count in the CSF should be normal and the protein content falling. Further lumbar punctures should be performed one year, eighteen months, two years and three years after the final course of treatment. Any evidence of renascent activity demands further vigorous treatment.

VIRUS INFECTIONS

Viruses are ultramicroscopic organisms dependent upon an intracellular existence. Acute infections cause the destruction of the host cell and oedema of the surrounding tissues. The reabsorption of oedema is responsible for the early functional improvement in these diseases. Subacute infections give rise to a typical amorphous structure inside the cell—an inclusion body. Viruses may lie dormant within the body only giving rise to symptoms when there is some extraneous irritation as sometimes happens in the cases of herpes (p. 120). Others are contagious and there is a recognizable pattern of infection, incubation period and signs. Although viruses may occasionally be isolated from the blood, and more frequently from the stool, the most reliable method of identification is by complement fixation tests. A sample of blood is taken as soon as the disease is suspected, and a second one six to eight weeks later. A positive diagnosis depends upon a rising titre.

The changes in the cerebrospinal fluid are not specific. In the acute phase of an illness there is frequently an increase in the cell count. For the first few days there may be a predominance of polymorphonuclear leucocytes, but an excess of lymphocytes is more typical. There may be a moderate rise in the protein content, but is seldom above 0·7 g/l and the sugar and chloride contents are unchanged.

Poliomyelitis

Acute anterior poliomyelitis most commonly occurs in epidemics. There are three distinct strains of virus (types, I, II, III), of which type I causes the greatest number of cases, but type II is the most virulent. Once established in the central nervous system, the virus causes the destruction of the anterior horn cells of the spinal cord and the cells of the brain-stem motor nuclei.

Infection most probably results from the ingestion of contaminated food or water. There is a delay of seven to fourteen days before the development of symptoms. During this time the virus becomes established in the bowel wall. Apart from a mild systemic upset the individual may not suffer any neurological disorder, and becomes a symptomless carrier. The virus is excreted in the faeces. This initial phase is sometimes accompanied by a viraemia and the patient experiences mild, flu-like symptoms. A few days later a second rise in temperature indicates invasion of the nervous system. It is thought that the virus reaches the spinal cord along the peripheral and autonomic nerves. This stage is accompanied by signs of meningeal irritation, headache, drowsiness, stiff neck and vomiting. The changes characteristic of a viral infection are found in the cerebrospinal fluid. Recovery may occur without the development of paralysis and the nature of the disorder will probably remain unrecognized unless there is a current epidemic.

In the **paralytic form** of poliomyelitis the onset of weakness occurs three to four dåys after the first signs of meningeal irritation. Deterioration may be expected during the next four days. The symptoms then remain static for ten to fourteen days after which improvement begins. This may continue for several months, but the bulk of useful recovery occurs in the first four months of the illness.

During the development of muscle weakness there is a generalized hypersensitivity, and the affected muscles are extremely tender. This is reminiscent of causalgia. The belief that the sympathetic nerve cells in the cord are affected, is borne out by the later development of skin changes and chilblains in the affected dermatomes.

The distribution of affected muscles is typically asymmetrical. The weakness is accompanied by wasting, hypotonia, fasciculation and diminished tendon reflexes. Involvement of the respiratory muscles or the muscles of deglutition poses special problems of nursing. There is no disturbance of sensation, and the patient remains fully conscious. Transient retention of urine may occur.

Treatment is based on the principle of resting the affected muscles as completely as possible. At the first sign of impaired respiratory function, a tracheostomy should be performed. Ventilation may then be assisted with an intermittent positive pressure respirator. When the acute phase of the illness has passed the patient is given graded exercises to strengthen the affected muscles. Any persisting weakness is corrected with appropriate calipers or splints.

Prophylaxis. Effective protection is provided by the Sabin oral vaccine. This is an attenuated live strain which causes a mild infection of the bowel and a subsequent immune response.

Late effects

Any persisting weakness will be accompanied by some muscle wasting and depression of related tendon reflexes. Fasciculation may be found many years after the initial attack. There are trophic changes in the affected limb. The skin is thin, the circulation is poor, and chilblains occur commonly. If growth is not complete at the time of the illness, the affected limb will remain shorter than its fellow.

Virus encephalitis

The virus of poliomyelitis may rarely cause an encephalitis, with cerebellar and upper motor neuron signs.

There was an epidemic of encephalitis lethargica soon after the first world war, but the only evidence of new cases since then is the sporadic occurrence of postencephalitic parkinsonism in young people. The brunt of the infection falls on the nuclei of the upper brain-stem, and results in disease of the basal ganglia, third nerve palsies, and various hypothalamic disorders.

Epidemic virus encephalitis occurs in different parts of the world, but is rare in the British Isles. Occasional cases are seen complicating mumps. The clinical picture is similar in all instances. There are usually signs of meningeal irritation, the patient complains of headache, he is drowsy, and coma develops sooner or later. Meningitis, polyneuritis or mononeuritis are common accompaniments. Some patients appear to benefit from steroid treatment if given at the onset of the disease. Betamethasone 4 mg four times a day is given for 4 days and then gradually withdrawn.

Herpes simplex has been recognized to be the cause of an acute *necrotizing encephalitis* most often affecting children and young adults. It presents with headache, vomiting, fits and abnormal behaviour. It progresses rapidly to confusion and coma. The temporal lobes are characteristically involved and the differential diagnosis is that for a space-occupying cerebral lesion.

The diagnosis is made by biopsy and immunofluorescence tests. It is commonly fatal but i.v. idoxuridine may be of benefit. Survivors have severe neurological deficits often associated with learning disorders, fits and permanent personality changes.

Herpes zoster

Herpes zoster (shingles) is a viral infection chiefly affecting the posterior root ganglia of the spinal cord or the sensory ganglia of the cranial nerves. A virus which is morphologically similar to that causing chicken pox has been identified in the skin vesicles, and patients with either disease show identical serological responses. Herpes zoster rarely occurs in childhood and it is suggested that the disease is due to a reactivation of the virus in a partially immune subject. Such reactivation may be caused by mechanical irritation of the nerve roots by tumour or one of the lymphomas.

The first symptoms are pain and reddening of the skin in the affected dermatome. Two or three days later there is an eruption of vesicles in the same area. The originally reddened skin darkens and the vesicles dry and separate, leaving white, anaesthetic scars.

One or two adjacent posterior root ganglia in the thoracic region are most commonly affected so that the pain, eruption and scarring occur in a band around one side of the trunk. Involvement of the first division of the trigeminal nerve may result in scarring of the cornea (ophthalmic herpes). Herpes of the geniculate ganglion (cranial nerve VII) causes an eruption in the external auditory canal and the throat and facial paralysis (p. 150).

The initial pain usually subsides as the dried crusts separate from the skin. Occasionally, and particularly in elderly people, the pain persists and becomes more severe. This is called post-herpetic neuralgia (p. 148).

Acute lymphocytic choriomeningitis

This is an acute, self-limiting, flu-like illness, characterized by signs of mild meningeal irritation, and an increase in the lymphocyte content of the cerebrospinal fluid. The disease is caused by a virus which is endemic in house mice. The patient is not seriously ill and requires no more than simple analgesics for the headache. He should be kept in bed until he is symptom free. If the illness persists for more than 10 days, if the patient is seriously ill, or if there are other signs of systemic or neurological disease, the diagnosis must be reconsidered. A lymphocytic meningeal reaction may accompany numerous neurological disorders including cerebral abscess, tuberculous meningitis, any of the virus infections of the central nervous system (e.g. poliomyelitis), syphilis and leptospirosis.

Chapter 16
Cerebrovascular Disease

Most of the symptoms described in this section are due to cerebral ischaemia. The high oxygen and nutritional requirements of the brain are reflected by the immediacy of symptoms if these supplies are restricted. Obstruction of the blood supply for a few minutes causes neuronal destruction.

Syncope (fainting)

Otherwise healthy people may be subject to brief episodes of cerebral ischaemia. These are often the result of imperfect venous return to the heart, for example, when standing still for long periods the blood becomes pooled in the legs. They also result from emotional shocks when a disturbance of neurovascular tone may be responsible. These attacks are called faints or syncope. The sufferer has a fairly long warning consisting of blurred vision, dizziness, yawning and weakness. He then slips limply to the floor, and if allowed to lie down he will recover in a few moments. He is pale and sweating and his pulse is of a small volume. If he is propped up during the faint, this will exaggerate the degree of cerebral hypotension; he may then convulse or be left with some permanent brain damage. Blurring of vision as an early symptom of cerebral ischaemia exemplifies the high oxygen requirements of the retinal ganglia. Prolonged arterial hypotension causes optic atrophy and blindness.

Arterial stenosis

Narrowing of the cranial arteries also causes ischaemia. Such narrowing (stenosis) may be due to one of the collagen vascular disorders, or syphilis, and this should be suspected in any young person presenting with evidence of cerebrovascular occlusion. Much more commonly it is caused by atherosclerosis. The aetiology of this condition is unknown. It consists of subintimal fatty deposits, upon which layers of thrombus may accumulate. The media of the vessel wall subsequently becomes thickened and unyielding. Hypertension and directional streaming of the blood within the arteries influence the sites at which atheroma develops. Atheromatous narrowing commonly occurs near the origin of the internal carotid artery (the carotid sinus) at its S-shaped bend in the cavernous sinus, and near the terminal bifurcation. The vertebral arteries and the basilar artery are frequently affected throughout their length.

Chronic cerebral ischaemia with numerous small infarcts leads to a progressive deterioration of brain function. This is called **cerebral arteriosclerosis.** Mental changes are usually prominent, including forgetfulness, particularly for recent events, querulousness and perseveration.

Strokes

Minor strokes or transient ischaemic attacks are probably due to the temporary lodgement of micro-emboli in the cerebral circulation. The emboli are accumulations of friable thrombus and platelets which originate on atheromatous plaques in the cranial arteries. The carotid sinus at the origin of the internal carotid artery is a common site for these plaques and the formation of emboli.

The attacks are characteristically short lived (less than 30 minutes) and may recur. They may consist of hemianaesthesia, hemiplegia, aphasia, vertigo, or loss of vision.

Such minor attacks are an indication of vascular disease, and often precede occlusion of a major vessel. The symptoms and signs of complete occlusion usually develop over a period of several hours.

The area supplied by the occluded vessel undergoes ischaemic necrosis (infarction). The tissues surrounding the infarction are at first oedematous, and it is the reabsorption of this oedema which accounts for much of the clinical improvement which occurs during the first few days after a cerebral thrombosis. Further improvement is slow and slight as there can be no functional recovery of an infarcted area of brain.

If facilities for CAT scanning are available this enables one to distinguish cerebral infarction from haemorrhage and oedema. In the completed stroke angiography is not indicated as surgical treatment is unlikely to be beneficial.

The extent and nature of the signs depends upon the individual vessel involved.

Occlusion of individual vessels

Internal carotid artery
Stenosis of the internal carotid artery commonly occurs at or near its origin in the neck. Its recognition is important as treatment may prevent crippling neurological symptoms.

Occlusion or stenosis of the internal carotid artery gives rise to a distinctive clinical presentation. The patient is likely to have one or more short-lived attacks of contralateral hemiparesis and ipsilateral uniocular blindness (Amaurosis fugax). This is due to ischaemia of the homolateral retina which receives its main arterial supply through the ophthalmic branch of the internal carotid artery. Even after a complete occlusion, the blindness due to retinal ischaemia usually recovers. This is because there is a well-developed anastomosis between the facial artery (from the external carotid system) and the ophthalmic artery. The leg often escapes involvement in the hemiplegia as the anterior cerebral artery is filled from the opposite side through the circle of Willis (p. 51). The presence of a carotid bruit, systemic hypertension and a history of clandication increase the likelihood that a significant stenosis will be found on angiography. This may be suitable for surgical treatment.

Anterior cerebral artery. Proximal to the medial striate branch, contralateral hemiplegia. Distal to the medial striate branch, contralateral paralysis with sparing of the arm and face.

Middle cerebral artery. Contralateral hemiplegia often sparing the leg, and hemianopia. Occlusion of the left middle cerebral artery also causes aphasia.

Posterior cerebral artery. Contralateral hemianopia.

Posterior inferior cerebellar artery. Vertigo. Ipsilateral ataxia. Contralateral spinothalamic sensory loss in the limbs and ipsilateral loss on the face. Nystagmus. Homolateral Horner's syndrome.

Basilar artery. Complete occlusion of the basilar artery is not compatible with life. Transient brain-stem ischaemia is common and results from stenosis of the vertebral or basilar arteries, or from kinking or compression of the vertebral arteries as they ascend through the cervical foramina.

Vertigo, diplopia, nystagmus, ataxia, loss of vision, hemiplegia or quadriplegia, loss or clouding of consciousness and akinetic attacks without unconsciousness, occur.

Treatment

The aim of treatment is to prevent the development of permanent neurological deficits. *Transient ischaemic attacks* deserve vigorous investigation. Hypertension should be controlled. Aspirin 300 mg daily lessens platelet stickiness and is a possible prophylactic. Anticoagulants are of uncertain value. After *infarction* the prognosis is poor if there is prolonged unconsciousness, dense hemiplegia, parietal lobe signs or loss of conjugate eye movements. Steroids may reduce oedema round an infarct. Early mobilization and rehabilitation is important. Prolonged rest in bed induces extension of the thrombosis, hypostatic pneumonia, bed sores and contractures.

Cerebral embolism

Strokes affecting young people without degenerative vascular disease are most often due to emboli complicating rheumatic heart disease. Thrombus develops on the scarred wall of a fibrillating left atrium. It becomes detached and because of the disposition of the vessels it is likely to lodge in a branch of the left middle cerebral artery. Hemiplegia unconsciousness or aphasia appear within seconds. To make this diagnosis there must be evidence of a source for the embolus. It is generally agreed that long-term anticoagulant therapy reduces the risk of further emboli. Additional therapy may be indicated for the underlying cardiac disease. The principles of early mobilization should be followed as in the cases of cerebral thrombosis.

Cerebral haemorrhage

Although dramatic, the onset of cerebral haemorrhage is not so acute as that of cerebral embolism and there is often a history of hypertension with its attendant symptoms.

There are seldom any specific prodromata such as the transient ischaemic attacks which precede the occlusion of a major vessel, but there may be a complaint of increasing headache and fatigue during the days preceding the haemorrhage. It often accompanies unusual physical effort or may be induced by an emotional crisis. It is unusual for an attack to come on during sleep and one might then suspect that the haemorrhage had occurred into a previously silent infarct. The signs develop over a period of a few minutes, and the disability becomes rapidly more extensive until consciousness is lost. During this time, the patient may complain of severe headache or on the other hand he may be unaware that anything is wrong.

The extravasation of blood into the cerebral tissue causes a sudden rise in intracranial pressure. Direct pressure and ischaemic changes in the brain-stem cause the loss of consciousness. In the majority of cases the source of haemorrhage is from the fine lenticulo-striate branches of the middle cerebral artery. The extruded blood bursts through the external capsule and the basal ganglia into the internal capsule causing hemiparesis. The paralysed limbs are at first flaccid due to neural shock. Within 24 hours an extensor plantar response can usually be obtained and tone returns within the next day or two. The patient may show signs of raised intracranial pressure and the entry of blood into the ventricular/subarachnoid space causes meningeal irritation with nuchal rigidity and uniform blood-staining of the cerebrospinal fluid.

Haemorrhage into the pons extends rapidly, causing widespread tissue destruction. The patient is deeply unconscious with bilateral paralysis of the face and limbs. His pupils are constricted and his temperature is raised.

The sudden release of blood tends to force the cerebral tissues apart rather than cause necrosis. Such a widespread dislocation of function often causes death within the first day or two without the recovery of consciousness. If the patient survives, the blood may become encapsulated to form a haemorrhagic cyst, or may be fully reabsorbed. If the blood is reabsorbed the lasting physical deficit may be quite small.

The recognition of a massive haemorrhage seldom presents any difficulty. A small localized haemorrhage may cause nothing more than a brief sensation of faintness, perhaps accompanied by numbness or weakness in one limb. This may easily be confused with an ischaemic episode. The dangers of anticoagulant therapy in such an instance are apparent. Occasionally there may be a progressive increase in the signs over several days so that a diagnosis of cerebral tumour is considered.

There has been a revival of interest in the surgical treatment of cerebral haemorrhage. The evacuation of a haematoma appears to benefit two groups of patients. (i) Those who after the ictus regain consciousness early but are left with a dense neurological deficit. (ii) Those who begin to improve but then show fluctuating signs. Angiography thus should be reserved for those patients who are not deeply unconscious and whose vital functions are not seriously affected.

Patients should be mobilized at the earliest opportunity. Severe hypertension should be treated with a hypotensive drug. Caution should be exercised in the reduction of blood pressure as a sudden drop may be attended by the occlusion of narrowed vessels. The patient should be advised to lead a temperate life avoiding excessive physical strain.

From this description it might be assumed that the differentiation of cerebrovascular accidents was easy. Sometimes the distinction between a cerebral haemorrhage and thrombosis is extremely difficult. If there is doubt then it is better to use the non-specific term 'stroke', than one which is speciously precise.

Subarachnoid haemorrhage

The presence of blood in the subarachnoid space may be due to head injury, the extension of an intracerebral haemorrhage, the rupture of an arteriovenous anomaly, or the rupture of an aneurysm. An **aneurysm** is the dilatation of an artery caused by the intima bulging through a defect in the media of the vessel wall. This may be secondary to acquired vascular disease but is more likely to be congenital. Although the majority of vascular accidents in young people may be attributed to this cause, subarachnoid haemorrhage occurs most commonly after the age of forty. Hypertension and increasing rigidity of the arterial tree are thus important additional factors.

Almost all intracranial aneurysms are found on the circle of Willis or its immediate branches (p. 51). The most important sites are the middle cerebral arteries (30 per cent), the anterior communicating artery (15 per cent) the basilar artery (15 per cent) and the internal carotid arteries (15 per cent). Eighty per cent of all aneurysms occur on the anterior half of the circle of Willis. They occur most commonly at the bifurcations or at the site of embryological branches. They are often associated with other vascular anomalies in the brain and elsewhere in the body. In 10 per cent of cases multiple aneurysms are found.

An enlarging aneurysm is never of sufficient size to cause an increase in the intracranial pressure but it may give rise to signs by local compression. An aneurysm on the internal carotid artery may compress the optic chiasm causing a nasal hemianopia, or an aneurysm of the posterior cerebral artery may damage the oculomotor nerve.

It is sometimes said that migraine may be a symptom of cerebral aneurysm. However, the incidence of aneurysm among migraine sufferers is no greater than it is in the rest of the population.

The **rupture of an aneurysm** usually accompanies physical exertion. Headache is the most prominent symptom. The onset is so acute that the patient often feels that he has been struck on the head. He may feel that something has burst inside his head (as indeed it has). There is often an immediate loss of consciousness, but unless the aneurysm ruptures into the tissue of the brain, there are no focal signs. Brain damage may complicate an aneurysm of the middle cerebral artery lying deep in the Sylvian fissure. Blood in the subarachnoid space causes meningeal irritation. Lumbar puncture immediately differentiates this condition from meningitis. It is important to distinguish the bloody cerebrospinal fluid of a subarachnoid haemorrhage from that due to a traumatic lumbar puncture. If the cerebrospinal fluid is blood stained, a few millilitres should be collected in three separate test tubes. If the staining is due to instrumental trauma, there will be a reduction in the amount of blood in the later tubes. If the bloodstained CSF is allowed to stand for half an hour, the red blood cells settle to the bottom of the tube, leaving the supernatant fluid colourless in the case of a recent traumatic puncture and xanthochromic (yellow) in the case of a subarachnoid haemorrhage of some hours' duration. The physical changes in the brain-stem which cause unconsciousness sometimes cause disturbance of metabolism, so that glucose and protein appear in the urine.

About a quarter of all patients with subarachnoid haemorrhage die without recovering consciousness. Of those who survive there is a real danger of further haemorrhage within the next six weeks. Once the diagnosis is made, the patient should be carefully nursed until consciousness is fully regained. Immediately after the rupture of the aneurysm the surrounding vessels go into spasm. This minimizes further haemorrhage. If angiography is undertaken too early, the residual spasm may obscure the site of an aneurysm.

Taking into consideration the patient's general condition, his level of consciousness and the presence or absence of shock, the majority of surgeons will choose to do angiography and operate at the earliest opportunity. Delay increases the incidence of recurrent haemorrhage. Treatment is aimed at direct occlusion of the aneurysm by open operation, or at reducing the arterial pressure to which it is exposed. This may be achieved by ligating the internal carotid artery in the neck. Should the patient survive beyond six weeks without active treatment, the likelihood of a recurrence decreases but the risk remains.

Arteriovenous anomaly

Although this lesion is also known as an angioma, it is not a neoplasm but a developmental malformation. It may occur in any part of the central nervous system but is most commonly found on the surface of the cerebral hemisphere in the distribution of the middle cerebral artery. It consists of a tangle of abnormal vessels within which there are numerous direct connections between the arterial and venous circulations. It is fed by one or more large arterial branches, and drained by wide venous channels.

Symptoms usually develop before the age of thirty and include headache, subarachnoid haemorrhage and epilepsy. The headache may be indistinguishable from idiopathic migraine. In such cases, the suspicion of underlying structural disease may be aroused by the prominence of physical signs during the aura, their persistence between attacks and the consistency with which one side of the body is affected. Subarachnoid haemorrhage is not the catastrophic event which accompanies the rupture of an aneurysm. The onset of symptoms is more gradual and the patient usually remains conscious. Focal epilepsy is the commonest clinical presentation of an arteriovenous malformation. Uncontrollable fits are the strongest indication for surgical treatment.

In a large proportion of cases a bruit may be heard over the site of the anomaly. Sometimes this is so loud that the patient can hear it himself. There may be signs of weakness, numbness or clumsiness in the contralateral limb.

The extent of the lesion can be demonstrated by angiography. Depending on its site, the surgeon may choose to excise the malformation or occlude the feeding vessels. Symptomatic treatment for the seizures will be required.

The risks of haemorrhage from an A-V anomaly increase during pregnancy and labour. Pregnancy should be advised against. The recognition of the anomaly during pregnancy is an indication for eventual Caesarian section.

Hypertensive encephalopathy

Severe hypertension, particularly if subject to paroxysmal rises may engender a dramatic sequence of neurological symptoms. These occur without any persisting macroscopic damage to the brain and are due to vascular spasm accompanied by acute cerebral oedema. It has been suggested that the arterial spasm is a protective response to sudden surges in blood pressure.

The episode presents with vomiting, headache, loss of consciousness and generalized convulsions. Almost all patients have papilloedema and the other fundal changes of severe hypertension. By definition, patients with hypertensive encephalopathy suffer no focal brain damage and exhibit no persisting focal signs. However, during a hypertensive crisis, dysphasia, hemiparesis and partial blindness may occur, and capillary haemorrhages may be found throughout the brain tissue.

Hypertensive encephalopathy requires emergency treatment. A parental hypotensive agent should be used, e.g. trimetaphan camsylate (Arfonad) 250 mg in 250 ml glucose/saline infusion. This ganglion blocker provides prompt short-term control of blood pressure. The rate of the drip is adjusted according to the patient's minute to minute response. The patient should be sedated with phenobarbitone 200 mg IM. Convulsions are best controlled with paraldehyde 10 ml IM. Betamethasone 4 mg tds, and frusemide may be given to reduce the cerebral oedema. Once the crisis is past, the patient should be maintained on an oral hypotensive agent.

THROMBOSIS OF THE CEREBRAL SINUSES

Thrombosis of the venous sinuses is most often a complication of infection, but aseptic thrombosis does occur.

Septic sinus thrombosis

The lateral sinus and the cavernous sinus are most often affected. *Thrombosis of the lateral sinus* is due to a spread of infection from the middle ear. If the ear infection is treated vigorously the presence of the thrombosed sinus may go unrecognized. The extension of septic thrombus into the jugular vein may involve the ninth, tenth and eleventh cranial nerves as they leave the skull through the jugular foramen.

Septic metastases from the face may reach the cavernous sinus through the anastomosis between the facial and ophthalmic veins. The cavernous sinus lies lateral to the body of the sphenoid. In its lateral wall run the internal carotid artery, the third, fourth and sixth cranial nerves, and the first and second division of the fifth nerve. *Thrombosis of the cavernous sinus* causes oedema of the face and orbital contents, paralysis of ocular movements and a burning pain about the eye. There may be numbness or hyperalgesia in the distribution of the ophthalmic and maxillary divisions of the fifth nerve. If neglected, the thrombosis will spread to the cavernous sinus of the opposite side.

Treatment with sulphonamides and penicillin have improved the prognosis in this condition.

Aseptic sinus thrombosis

Aseptic thrombosis of the dural sinuses results from increased coagulability of the blood. This occurs during the puerperium and in pneumococcal pneumonia. Gross dehydration, inanition, and cachexia also predispose to thrombosis. Thus, infants in the first year of life and the elderly are especially vulnerable. Venous sinus thrombosis sometimes complicates head injury.

The superior sagittal sinus is most often affected. The obstruction of venous drainage raises the capillary pressure, causes a degree of cerebral oedema, and increases the formation of cerebrospinal fluid in the choroid plexus. Furthermore the reabsorption of CSF is hindered if the arachnoid granulations are involved in the thrombosis. There is a consequent rise in the intracranial pressure causing headache and vomiting, but consciousness is usually retained. If the thrombosis extends to the cortical veins, weakness of the legs and focal motor seizures may occur.

Benign intracranial hypertension

This is also known as pseudotumour cerebri. A few of these cases are secondary to thrombosis of the dural venous sinuses, but in the majority the aetiology remains obscure. It is commonest in women in their thirties or forties of stout build, who have recently been pregnant. There is also a recognized association with the menarche. The patient complains of persistent headache and vomiting. Apart from papilloedema, ocular palsies are the only common sign. Fits and mental deterioration do not occur. Computerized axial tomography shows that there is no displacement of intracranial structures and that the ventricles are of normal or small size.

Although this is a benign condition there is a danger that longstanding papilloedema will cause optic atrophy. Repeated lumbar punctures may induce a remission but otherwise frusemide or betamethasone 8–12 mg daily should be used. In refractory cases or if the visual acuity deteriorates, neurosurgical assistance should be sought.

Chapter 17
Organic Dementia

Dementia is a disorder of all the mental processes. It is characterized by changes in the subject's personality and by deterioration in his memory and reasoning ability. The memory loss is most profound for recent events. Distant memory seems good by comparison, but careful questioning reveals considerable lacunae. The patient becomes careless of his personal condition and there may be emotional outbursts often foreign to his character. There are wide swings of mood, and the patient is given to morbid rumination. Such deterioration is part of the natural course of senescence. It is thought to be due to chronic cerebral anoxia secondary to arteriosclerosis.

The appearance of dementia in middle age demands thorough investigation as some of the causative conditions are amenable to treatment. The disorders which should be considered in the differential diagnosis are:
1. The deficiency diseases.
2. Metabolic disorders.
3. Cerebral tumour.
4. General paralysis of the insane.
5. Head injury.
6. Epilepsy.
7. Huntington's chorea.
8. Normal pressure hydrocephalus.
9. The 'presenile dementias'.

Dementia is essentially subacute or chronic. An acute mental disorder complicating organic brain disease is termed *delirium*. This occurs in some of the deficiency diseases, such as Wernicke's encephalopathy, during the acute phase of encephalitis, or complicating metabolic disorders. It is characterized by restlessness, irritability, disorientation and hallucinations. Such symptoms of acute illness may precede the appearance of dementia or be superimposed upon the established syndrome.

(1) The deficiency diseases

Organic mental disorders may accompany the other neurological symptoms due to deficiencies of thiamine, nicotinic acid and vitamin B12. Deficiencies of thiamine and nicotinic acid cause peripheral neuritis and a relatively acute delirium. The delirium due to thiamine deficiency is known as *Wernicke's encephalopathy*. Haemorrhages occur in the upper brain-stem, especially in the region of the mammillary bodies. Third and fourth nerve palsies are common. There is a profound memory disturbance which particularly affects the patient's ability to place events in their correct time relationship. Being at a loss he may confabulate to fill the gaps in his recollections. Deficiencies of thiamine are responsible for most of the symptoms of chronic alcoholism and hyperemesis of pregnancy. Immediate treatment with thiamine (vitamin B1) causes a rapid improvement in the neurological signs and a progressive recovery from the dementia. Thiamine treatment is a valuable first aid measure in any undiagnosed dementia and its effect does not obscure other possible diagnoses.

The onset of dementia associated with vitamin B12 deficiency (p. 163) is insidious. The symptoms of neuropathy and cord disease may be slight and easily overlooked. There is usually a typical megaloblastic anaemia but dementia can develop with a normal peripheral blood picture. Serum vitamin B12 levels are low or zero. Treatment with parenteral B12 brings about a rapid and spectacular improvement. This should not be used as a therapeutic test.

(2) Metabolic disorders
1 Repeated or prolonged episodes of hypoglycaemia cause neuronal dysfunction and degeneration. There is usually a history of altered consciousness, feelings of faintness or periods of mental confusion.
2 Hypothyroidism causes a slowing of mental function which will progress to overt dementia if left untreated.
3 Chronic liver disease may cause a fluctuant dementia and a coarse tremor of the hands.

(3) Cerebral tumour
A prefrontal cerebral tumour may present with mental changes, but no other physical signs or symptoms. Tumours at this site do not cause raised intracranial pressure. Tremor and a grasp reflex are sometimes found. Electroencephalography may help in locating the lesion and neuroradiological studies are usually diagnostic.

(4) General paralysis of the insane
General paresis is usually accompanied by the stigmata of neurosyphilis (p. 116). A positive FTA and active cerebrospinal fluid confirm the diagnosis.

(5) Head injury
A severe head injury accompanied by prolonged unconsciousness is likely to be associated with mental changes. The gradual development of mental disorder in an elderly patient, weeks or months after a head injury, should alert one to the possibility of a subdural

haematoma. It is often accompanied by fluctuating drowsiness, headache and weakness of the limbs.

2 Repeated lesser injuries, such as are suffered by professional boxers, commonly result in dementia, tremor and seizures—the punch drunk syndrome.

(6) Epilepsy
Poorly controlled epileptics frequently show some degree of dementia. This may be due to the repeated hypoxic episodes, the predisposing condition, or the result of intoxication with anticonvulsants.

(7) Huntington's chorea
A familial disease consisting of gross choreic movements, facial grimacing and a staggering gait. Uncommonly, the dementia may precede the development of involuntary movement (p. 141).

(8) Normal pressure hydrocephalus
An uncommon condition sometimes attributed to a preceding head injury. An impaired circulation of CSF over the convexity of the brain leads to increasing ventricular dilatation and dementia. There is a characteristic association of dementia with urinary incontinence and an unsteady gait. Intracranial monitoring confirms the diagnosis and is a usual prerequisite for surgical treatment.

(9) 'Presenile dementia'—Alzheimer's and Pick's diseases
These are pathological diagnoses. The former is applied to a generalized cerebral atrophy while the latter is reserved for atrophy limited to the frontal and temporal lobes. These are diagnoses which should be made only by exclusion. Clinically the two cannot be differentiated with any certainty and the exercise is unrewarding. There is no treatment.

Seven steps in the *investigation* of dementia in middle age.
 1. Detailed history from the patient and from a reliable member of his family. This must include a full family history.
 2. A complete neurological and general examination.
 3. FTA (absorbed).
 4. Radio isotope scanning.
 5. Serum vitamin B12.
 6. Electroencephalography.

7. Computerized axial tomography of the skull.
8. Examination of the cerebrospinal fluid.

Chapter 18
Diseases of the Basal Ganglia

PARKINSONISM

Parkinsonism is a syndrome encompassing a generalized poverty of movement, tremor and rigidity. It is due to a functional imbalance of the cerebral neurotransmitters with a relative deficiency of dopamine. Occurring spontaneously, it is a progressive degenerative disorder of the basal ganglia predominantly affecting the substantia nigra. Similar symptoms are induced by certain neuroleptic drugs which deplete the brain of dopamine or block its uptake in the pallidum.

Postencephalitic parkinsonism is now uncommon. Those rare cases of juvenile parkinsonism deserve full investigation so that a potentially treatable condition is not neglected.

Idiopathic parkinsonism

This is a disease of late middle age (45–60 years) affecting men and women equally. The first and often the most prominent symptom is *tremor*. At the onset this is intermittent and may appear only when the patient is tired. It most often affects one hand, spreading to the leg on the same side and later to the other limbs. The jaw and tongue are commonly involved but not the head. There is an alternating contraction of agonists and antagonists, the rate is slow, 3–6 beats per second, and hand movements are affected before the rest of the arm. It is most prominent when the limbs are at rest although it subsides during sleep. It can be suppressed by vigorous voluntary movements, but it seriously interferes with delicate precise movements such as holding a cup or using a knife and fork. Less apparent than the static tremor is a fine action tremor. Its frequency is from six to twelve cycles per second and unlike the static tremor it is unidirectional. Each jerk is in the direction of the chosen target.

Rigidity usually follows the same distribution as the tremor. A greater effort is required for any voluntary movement as it must be made against actively contracting antagonists and without the aid of the synergists. The patient interprets this as a primary weakness and he fatigues rapidly. The resistance to passive movement may be smooth throughout its range (plastic rigidity) or intermittent (cog-wheel rigidity). Rigidity is often accompanied by pain in the muscles, particularly those of the limb girdles and the trunk. Such discomfort often gives rise to a distressing restlessness.

In addition to the slowness resulting from rigidity, there is a general retardation of voluntary movement called *bradykinesia*. It is difficult for the patient to initiate movements, to vary his posture or to supplement willed movements with unconsciously generated supportive movements. It may be seen in the patient's difficulty in rising from a chair, in starting to walk, speak or write. Speech is slowed and often slurred. His writing is small and cramped, and becomes even smaller as he continues. The patient does not swing his arms when walking, his face is expressionless and his voice is unmodulated. Due to a disorder of the normal pattern of swallowing, saliva gathers and drips from the half-open mouth.

Postural disturbances result in an increasing stoop, and the patient stands with his head bent and his arms flexed in front of his body. He takes short steps and may break into a shuffling run to maintain his balance.

Physical examination shows that in spite of the apparent weakness the muscle power is not reduced. The deep tendon reflexes are normal and the plantar responses are flexor. Sensation is normal. Special investigations show no significant abnormalities.

Progressive supranuclear palsy is a symptom complex comprising a parkinsonlike illness, dementia and a failure of upward gaze. In the *Shy-Drager* syndrome, parkinsonism and postural hypotension occur together.

Treatment
There is an imbalance between inhibitory influences mediated by dopamine and facilitatory influences mediated by acetylcholine. The imbalance may be restored by supplementing the dopamine or using an anticholinergic drug.

(a) **Levodopa.** Oral dopamine will not cross the blood–brain barrier; its precursor levodopa (l-dopa) will. While still in the peripheral circulation much of the l-dopa is metabolized to dopamine, noradrenaline and adrenaline. A decarboxylase inhibitor can be combined with l-dopa (Sinemet, Madopar) to slow its metabolism and make more l-dopa available in the brain.

Three quarters of parkinsonian patients benefit from l-dopa. It is especially effective in relieving bradykinesia. The drug should be given initially in small doses and gradually built up. Side effects include nausea, depression and dyskinesia (see below). Prolonged treatment is complicated by the on/off phenomenon; sudden, severe yet transient bradykinesia. Avoid the concurrent use of monoamine oxidase inhibitors (risk of dangerous hypertension) and pyridoxine.

(b) The **anticholinergic drugs.** The naturally occurring solanaceous drugs are now not often used, and the synthetic spasmolytics have similar side effects which limit their use. These include dryness of the mouth, blurring of vision (due to paralysis of accommodation) and constipation. Hallucinations, confusional states and nightmares sometimes result from their use in elderly patients. More seriously, they may also cause urinary retention or glaucoma. They give some relief from rigidity and pain but have much less effect on tremor and scarcely any on bradykinesia.

The doses quoted below are those contained in the standard tablets. The regime for all of these drugs is the same. The patient is given one tablet twice a day and then the dose is gradually increased until the symptoms are relieved or the side effects become intolerable.

Benzhexol HCl (Artane), 2 mg.
Procyclidine HCl (Kemadrin), 5 mg.
Benztropine methane sulphonate (Cogentin), 2 mg.
Orphenadrine HCl (Disipal), 50 mg.

(c) Other drugs. Amantidine hydrochloride is beneficial but seems to lose its effectiveness. Bromocriptine has a similar effect to l-dopa.

Drug-induced movement disorders

Some neuroleptic drugs induce extrapyramidal symptoms. Phenothiazines and butyrophenones block the uptake of dopamine in the pallidum; reserpine and tetrabenazine deplete the brain of dopamine. These mechanisms result in a syndrome indistinguishable from parkinsonism. It is relieved by dose reduction or the addition of an anticholinergic drug. The use of phenothiazines and butyrophenones may be complicated by the development of *dyskinesias*. These include:

1. Acute dystonic reaction: usually in young people in the first days of treatment. Discontinue the neuroleptic and give an anticholinergic IV.

2. Akathisia: restless tic-like movements.

3. Tardive dyskinesia: delayed onset, in elderly subjects. Difficult to treat. Withdrawal of drug may worsen symptoms or provoke them.

Dyskinesias, twisting movements of the extremities and facial grimacing complicate the use of l-dopa in parkinsonism. This is possibly due to heightened sensitivity of the damaged neurons.

Wilson's disease

Wilson's disease (hepato-lenticular degeneration) is an uncommon condition characterized by cirrhosis of the liver, and a neurological syndrome consisting of rigidity and tremor. Its recognition is important in that further deterioration can be halted, and in some cases, reversed by appropriate treatment. It affects both sexes and usually manifests itself before the age of twenty. It is an inherited disorder and clinically unaffected siblings may bear the trait. There is an inability to form the copper-globulin complex, caeruloplasmin. The serum copper instead of being firmly bound to the globulin, circulates in a freely available form. It is deposited in the brain and liver and an excessive amount of copper also appears in the urine (more than 100 micromols/day). The basal ganglia have a special affinity for copper and there is a consequent destruction of these neurons. The neurological symptoms consist of rigidity and tremor with an additional element of athetosis. The severely affected patient is dysarthric and his face is set in an open-mouthed fatuous smile. Mental deterioration is usually progressive. There may be no clinical signs of liver disease, or the patient may be deeply jaundiced and show evidence of advanced hepatic cirrhosis. If present, the Kayser–Fleischer ring is pathognomonic. This is a smoky yellow-brown deposit seen round the edge of the cornea, in front of the iris.

The diagnosis is confirmed by finding a greatly reduced serum copper oxidase activity, or excess copper in the urine.

Treatment with penicillamine (600–900 mg/day) mobilizes and binds the copper which is excreted in the urine. This must be continued indefinitely and the ideal dose is that which maintains the highest excretion of copper in the urine. As the copper deposits become depleted it is usually possible to reduce the dose of penicillamine to a maintenance level of 150 mg three times a day. The drugs used in the symptomatic treatment of parkinsonism (p. 138) may be of value for the relief of tremor and rigidity.

Congenital athetosis

This is one form of cerebral palsy and the aetiology of these conditions was discussed on p. 95. The whole spectrum of involuntary movements may be seen and the severity varies from mild restlessness to continuous and extensive choreo-athetoid contortions. It is present from birth, but the movements may only become apparent when the child begins to develop postural control. The athetosis may be an isolated phenomenon or associated with paraplegia, diplegia, mental retardation or seizures.

Kernicterus

Kernicterus results from haemolytic disorder of intrauterine life usually a complication of Rh and ABO incompatibility between the mother and the fetus. Infants with severe kernicterus die soon after birth, and the post-mortem examination shows extensive neuronal degeneration in the basal ganglia. Survivors often show serious mental retardation. Milder forms of kernicterus are compatible with normal life but affected individuals may present in childhood or early adulthood with ataxia and choreo-athetoid movements.

Chorea

Chorea is a term which describes sudden, jerky movements of the limbs, which although not fully co-ordinated sometimes have the appearance of purposefulness. The power of the limb is normal to clinical testing, although the tone is reduced and the reflexes are commonly pendular.

Diseases of the Basal Ganglia

Sydenham's chorea is a benign disorder of childhood and one of the manifestations of rheumatic fever. Characteristically the other signs of rheumatism are quite slight. In addition to the jerking movements of the limbs, the child makes smirking grimaces and the emotional disturbances which frequently accompany the neurological disease may obscure its true physical nature. The disorder is self-limiting and responds to mild sedatives such as phenobarbitone 30 mg twice a day.

Huntington's chorea is a progressive disorder consisting of dementia and bizarre involuntary movements. It is inherited as a dominant characteristic and usually first appears in middle age. Less commonly it may occur in childhood. Neuronal degeneration is widespread throughout the brain and the cells of the basal ganglia are particularly affected. Pneumoencephalography shows a characteristic dilatation of the lateral ventricles where their walls overlie the normal convexity of the caudate nuclei.

An apparent restlessness of the limbs is commonly the first manifestation of the disease. The gait has a curious springiness, but as the illness progresses the violence of the involuntary movement makes the patient stagger as though drunk. Facial grimacing is prominent. Mental deterioration occurs sooner or later (p. 133). Tetrabenzine 10 mg three or four times a day is effective in controlling the involuntary movements; overdosage with this drug induces a parkinson-like syndrome.

Tremor may occur as an isolated symptom. It is sometimes familial or may occur sporadically in elderly people. It commonly affects the head in contrast with the tremor of parkinsonism. Propranolol 80–120 mg daily is an effective treatment.

Chapter 19
Headache

Headache is a common symptom which may be of trivial origin or the expressions of serious disease.

There are several well-recognized mechanisms to which headache may be attributed and each has a typical symptomatology. Patients seldom consult their doctors until the headache has become chronic. By this time it has been the object of considerable introspection and the clinical features have become blurred. Diagnosis is correspondingly more difficult.

Not all of the intracranial structures are pain sensitive. The meninges of the anterior and posterior fossa, the venous sinuses, the major arteries, the falx and tentorium cerebelli are supplied with fibres carrying pain sensation to the fifth, ninth and tenth cranial nerves. The parenchyma of the brain is insensitive to normally painful stimuli.

Vascular headache
This is a throbbing headache. It is caused by the dilatation of the major intracranial or extracranial vessels and the consequent stretching of the pain sensitive fibres in their walls. Dilatation of the intracranial arteries is a common response to circulating toxins, e.g. accompanying fever or in the post-alcoholic hang-over. The headache is worsened by shaking the head or stooping, and its cause is usually apparent. The headache of migraine is caused by the dilatation of the extracranial arteries.

Meningeal irritation
This is a persistent, non-throbbing, often severe headache which is associated with neck stiffness. It is caused by the introduction of a foreign irritant substance into the subarachnoid space. Examples of such substances are blood (subarachnoid haemorrhage), the products of infection (meningitis) and air (pneumoencephalography).

Tumour headache
The headache is dull, poorly localized, non-throbbing and worsened

by change of posture. It often appears soon after waking in the morning to lessen later in the day. It is caused by displacement of the pain sensitive intracerebral structures. Such displacement may be sufficient to cause a rise in the intracranial pressure, when papilloedema will be found.

Referred headache
Painful conditions affecting extracranial structures may cause referred headache. The investigation of a patient with headache should include examination of the following organs:
    Orbits: pain of glaucoma.
    Nasopharynx: nasopharyngeal carcinoma.
    Sinuses: sinusitis.
    Ear: otitis media.
    Mouth: dental caries.
    Temporal arteries: arteritis.
    Cervical spine: spondylosis.

Tension headache
A diagnosis of tension headache should be made only when the physical examination has failed to reveal any significant abnormality. Headache is often only one of many complaints. It tends to persist for weeks or months although it rarely interferes with sleep. It is commonly described as having a crushing or pressing quality or likened to a tight band round the head. It is seldom relieved by analgesics.

A worried, anxious patient may also have physical disease.

MIGRAINE

Migraine is a syndrome characterized by periodic hemicranial headache associated with prostration and vomiting. In the majority of cases, migraine is idiopathic, that is, it arises from no recognizable structural disorder. A small minority are, however, symptomatic of some underlying disease. Migraine appearing for the first time in middle age should rouse the suspicion of a symptomatic origin, particularly if symptoms or signs persist between attacks. Intracranial aneurysm, angioma and arteritis are occasionally responsible. Angiography is the only certain way of identifying symptomatic migraine.

Idiopathic migraine usually develops in adolescence or before the age of thirty. There is commonly a family history of headaches, and the patient himself may have suffered from travel sickness or 'biliousness' in childhood. He is typically conscientious and ambitious, but perhaps lacking the drive or ability to execute his schemes. The onset of migraine can sometimes be dated from the assumption of new responsibilities or a period of physical or emotional stress. Individual attacks often develop on the day following physical or mental fatigue, so that a weekend, or the first day of a holiday, is spoiled. A woman may experience attacks at the time of menstruation and the tendency is then likely to subside after the menopause. The frequency of attacks varies from two or three times a week to two or three times in a lifetime.

The patient is usually aware that an attack is impending. He may feel listless and short-tempered or find that normal intensities of light, noise and odour are difficult to tolerate. Not infrequently, the onset of an attack is marked by an aura. Visual auras are common. These may consist of fading or wavering of the vision or the more dramatic teichopsia. The patient is first aware of a bright scintilla just lateral to the point of fixation. This expands as an arc of flickering brilliance which gradually fills one-half of the visual field. A scotoma of varying density spreads over the same part of the visual field.

This phase of the attack is due to arterial constriction and consequent cerebral or retinal ischaemia. The cause of the vasoconstriction is unknown. Unilateral numbness, weakness and dysphasia are less common types of aura. The aura usually lasts from five to twenty minutes after which the function returns. The headache then ensues. This is at first hemicranial and often starts above or behind the eye. It expands over one side of the head and later may affect both sides. It is a severe throbbing 'vascular' headache. The patient is acutely miserable, photophobic and nauseated. Vomiting commonly occurs, sometimes heralding the end of an attack.

During a severe attack the superficial cranial vessels are dilated and the temporal artery can be seen pulsating. The face is suffused, the mucosae of the nose congested, and the eye runs with tears. It is thought that the pain is due to vasodilatation which stretches the pain sensitive fibres in the vessel walls. Compression of the temporal artery sometimes relieves the headache temporarily.

The headache lasts from four to twelve hours, often subsiding during sleep. In some instances the headache may last for three or four days at a time. Fluid retention may play a part in the causation of the headache, as there is sometimes a brisk diuresis at the end of an attack. On the following day some patients feel tired while others feel curiously elated.

The headache and the aura may occur on the same or opposite sides. Paradoxically the headache and aura may concide. The syndrome is frequently incomplete so that the aura and sometimes the headache is not experienced. It is probable that the majority of unexplained paroxysmal headaches are due to this mechanism, particularly if there is a strong family history of headaches.

Thrombosis in a constricted artery resulting in cerebral infarction is a rare complication. Thrombosis in a retinal artery may occur but is also uncommon. The basilar artery is sometimes involved in the vasoconstriction giving rise to vertigo, faintness and ophthalmoplegia (ophthalmoplegic migraine). If the diplopia persists for more than two or three hours the possibility that it is due to an arterial aneurysm must be considered.

Treatment

An attempt should be made to define any factor which might precipitate an attack. It may then be possible for the patient to re-order his life so that these situations are avoided. Certain foods, such as cocoa, cheese, citrus fruit and strongly flavoured alcoholic drinks may act as triggers. Manipulation of the environment is usually impossible and recourse is made to symptomatic treatment; the simplest and least toxic drug being the first choice.

Soluble aspirin: 0·6 to 1·0 g is sufficient for mild and infrequent attacks.

A tranquillizer may be appropriate for the tense patient. The use of prophylactics should be reserved for the patient whose life is being disrupted by frequent attacks.

Pizotifen 0·5–1·0 mg, 3 times a day.

Prochlorperazine 5–15 mg, 3 times a day.

Propranolol 10 mg, 3 times a day.

Ergotamine tartrate: this drug causes vasoconstriction and if taken early in an attack will prevent the development of headache. It is best given by subcutaneous injection, 0·5 mg. Suppositories are an efficient and increasingly popular method of administration. Sublingual tablets are the least effective presentation. A measured dose of ergotamine tartrate may be delivered as an aerosol (Medihaler) which is inhaled and absorbed from the respiratory tract and lungs. Dihydroergotamine (1 mg tablets), two tablets may be taken at the beginning of an attack and it is sometimes used as a prophylactic. Ergotamine is contraindicated in the presence of degenerative vascular disease. The prescribed dose should not be exceeded.

Caffeine citrate: 0·5 g. This is often effective in the treatment of those patients who suffer disconcerting symptoms attributable to the vasoconstrictive phase, without any subsequent headache.

Chapter 20
Facial Pain

The patient generally can differentiate headache, which he feels inside his head, from facial pain which he recognizes as being superficial. Persistent facial pain may be due to disease of the skin, the subcutaneous tissues, muscle, sinuses, teeth and arteries.

Temporal arteritis (giant cell arteritis) causes severe persistent pain localized in the temporal artery. It occurs in the elderly, and men are more often affected than women. There is bluish discoloration of the skin over the artery, which is swollen, tender and non-pulsating. There may be evidence of arteritis elsewhere in the body. The retinal vessels are commonly affected and involvement of the central artery of the retina causes blindness. There is evidence of generalized systemic upset, with fever, leucocytosis and a raised sedimentation rate. Treatment with ACTH or high doses of corticosteroids should be started immediately to lessen the chance of blindness. The reduction in the dose of steroids is guided by the ESR. Biopsy of the swollen vessel provides histological confirmation of the diagnosis and relieves the pain.

Nasopharyngeal carcinoma also causes severe constant pain. There is early metastasis to the lymph nodes of the neck, and the tumour may be palpated directly by hooking the finger over the back of the soft palate. A lateral X-ray of the skull may show a mass in the nasopharynx.

Trigeminal neuralgia is the name given to brief paroxysms of searing facial pain. It occurs in the elderly without any accompanying physical signs. In younger people it may be symptomatic of structural disease such as disseminated sclerosis. In this instance some evidence of sensory depression is often found in the distribution of the trigeminal nerve.

The pain is felt as an agonizing stab originating in a trigger spot, and radiating into the rest of the affected division. The second and third divisions are most frequently involved and the trigger spots lie around the mouth and nose. Touching one of the spots is usually sufficient to provoke an attack. The initial pain lasts for two or three seconds and is followed by a dull, burning sensation in the same distribution. It is usual for these attacks to come in bouts, lasting for a few weeks or months at a time. During such a period, paroxysm will be precipitated by the slightest stimulus such as a touch or a breath of wind on the face. The patient becomes afraid to eat, drink, speak, wash or shave. Attacks of pain seldom occur during sleep. This seems to be the result of a generalized depression of neuronal excitability, and it may explain the success of anticonvulsants in the treatment of this condition.

A considerable proportion of patients respond well to carbamazepine (Tegretol). One tablet is given twice a day initially, and the dose is gradually increased until the pain is relieved or intolerable side effects occur. Like other anticonvulsants, this drug may depress the function of the bone marrow. Some neurologists favour injection of alcohol into the affected branches of the nerve, where they leave the skull.

More permanent relief is obtained by sectioning the sensory fibres proximal to the trigeminal ganglion in Meckel's cave. This operation can be performed on the most debilitated patients with little danger. If the first division of the nerve is not involved, these fibres can be spared. If ophthalmic fibres must be sectioned, then some form of protection will be necessary for the anaesthetic cornea on that side. Radiofrequency thermocoagulation can be used to destroy the pain-sensitive fibres in the trigeminal ganglion selectively, preserving the sense of touch.

The central fibres of the trigeminal nerve are often involved in medullary lesions. Thus facial pain may be a prominent feature of disseminated sclerosis and thrombosis of the posterior inferior cerebellar artery. In these cases it is usually accompanied by impaired sensation on the face.

Migrainous neuralgia (histaminic cephalgia)
Attacks of migrainous neuralgia also come in bouts, each lasting for several weeks. The middle-aged patient experiences an attack every night during this time. It wakens him from sleep between 2 a.m. and 5 a.m. The pain is localized about one eye. The surrounding skin is suffused, swollen and tender. The pain lasts from 15 to 30 minutes and then resolves completely. There is no aura and the patient is not nauseated. No physical abnormality can be detected on examination. It responds to ergotamine tartrate 0·5 mg by subcutaneous injection, and sometimes to the oral preparation. It has been recommended that this should be given on retiring, for six days in the week. On the seventh day the patient should go without treatment to see whether or not a remission has occurred.

Post-herpetic neuralgia
Post-herpetic neuralgia is a persistent, severe burning pain at the site of a previous herpetic eruption. It is precipitated by the slightest stimulus. The patient is nearly always elderly and the intensity of the pain is such as to make his life a burden. This may result in addiction to opiates, depression and suicide. There is usually a clear-cut history of shingles (p. 120) and scarring of the skin is apparent.

Treatment is difficult. Various forms of physical therapy have been used including vibratory massage, percussive sprays and superficial radiotherapy over the affected area. A combination of analgesics and a thymoleptic may bring some relief, and carbamazepine is sometimes effective. Transcutaneous electrical stimulation is worthy of a trial. Section of the affected nerve root is of no value.

Paget's disease of the skull often gives rise to local pain and tenderness. The bone pain is burning in quality and persistent.

Psychogenic facial pain is common and causes great distress. Its recognition and satisfactory treatment is a major challenge to the physician. Not infrequently it is a presenting symptom of depression and it may respond to antidepressive therapy. As in the case of those other symptoms attributable to mental disorder, a careful physical examination is necessary to exclude structural disease.

Chapter 21
Facial Palsy

Facial paralysis may occur as part of a generalized disorder such as the Guillain-Barré syndrome or motor neuron disease. It may complicate intracranial lesions as sometimes happens with an acoustic nerve tumour, and it may appear as an isolated benign condition.

The cause of this benign unilateral facial paralysis, **Bell's Palsy**, is unknown, although it is popularly attributed to sitting in a draught. From the course of this illness it seems likely that oedema of the nerve sheath compresses the nerve as it traverses the narrow facial canal. It may be secondary to a virus infection, and it affects young and old alike.

The paralysis is often first apparent on waking, and usually worsens during the next few hours. The onset is accompanied by a dull ache felt behind the ear and spreading into the face. The patient may describe the weakness as a feeling of woodenness or numbness, but sensory testing is always normal. As it is a lower motor neuron lesion the muscles of both the upper and lower parts of the face are affected. It is often impossible for the patient to close his eyes completely and an attempt to do so results in the eyeball rolling upwards (Bell's phenomenon). His mouth is drawn over by the actively contracting muscles on the opposite side of the face; saliva may dribble from his mouth and food gathers between the cheek and gum. It is uncommon for both sides of the face to be affected simultaneously.

If the nerve is affected in the proximal part of the facial canal (Fig. 26), then the intermediate nerve of Wrisberg and the nerve to stapedius will be involved. The former results in a loss of taste sensation over the anterior two-thirds of the tongue. Lesions of the nerve to stapedius cause hyperacusis, that is, sudden variations in the apparent loudness of sounds.

The oedema subsides within seven to ten days. If any recovery has begun within this period then it is likely to be fairly complete. If there is no apparent recovery, then the measurement of strength/duration curves is a valuable aid to prognosis. A normal curve indicates a likelihood of recovery, while a degeneration curve suggests that no recovery is likely to occur. Full recovery may be delayed for five to ten weeks.

Treatment

Facial pain should be treated with an analgesic. If steriods are given within the first two or three days of the onset of the illness, the rate and degree of recovery will be greater. As soon as the pain subsides the patient should be instructed in facial exercises which he performs in front of a mirror for at least ten minutes, three times a day. If he is unable to close his eye, he should be provided with a shield to prevent damage to the cornea. Bland drops should be instilled several times a day. A drooping face should be supported with a piece of (transparent) adhesive tape. Although recovery is the rule, this may not be complete, and a light acrylic splint for the corner of the mouth will improve the cosmetic effect.

Herpes of the geniculate ganglion of the facial nerve also causes facial paralysis. The onset is accompanied by the much more severe herpetic pain and a vesicular eruption in the external auditory canal and behind the ear. The recovery of facial movement after geniculate herpes is complete in about a half of the cases.

Facial paralysis not uncommonly occurs as a symptom of *disseminated sclerosis*.

Chapter 22
Labyrinthine Vertigo

In an acute vestibular disturbance the patient tends to fall towards the affected labyrinth when standing or walking; the fast phase of nystagmus is away from the affected side.

Ménière's disease is manifest by recurrent paroxysmal vertigo associated with progressive cochlear deafness. It is a disorder of middle age and affects men more often than women. The immediate cause of this disorder seems to be a distension of the membranous labyrinth due to excess secretion of endolymph. The reason for this is unknown and has been variously ascribed to hyperaemia, allergy and a generalized electrolyte disturbance.

The attacks vary in severity from a mild feeling of unsteadiness to vertigo of such violence that the patient is thrown to the ground. The vestibular disturbance is often preceded by a deafness for high notes. This is accompanied by high-pitched tinnitus. During an acute attack, the tinnitus becomes louder and often of a lower pitch. The attacks of vertigo occur at varying intervals. Several may occur together during which time the patient experiences a feeling of fullness in his head.

The onset of an attack is typically acute. Vertigo, unsteadiness, nausea, sweating, vomiting and an increase in the deafness and tinnitus are prominent. The patient usually lies still on the ground or in bed unwilling to move for fear of provoking further vertigo. There is no loss of consciousness. There is a rhythmical nystagmus with the fast phase away from the affected ear. The acute stage of the attack lasts from 15 minutes to 2 hours. On recovery, any sudden or unusual movement may still provoke transient vertigo.

The tuning fork tests indicate a nerve type of deafness on the same side as the tinnitus. The recruitment test (p. 71) shows a recruiting deafness which differentiates Ménière's disease from lesions of the auditory nerve. The deafness is progressive, but when it is complete the attacks of vertigo subside.

In the acute attack the patient should be given chlorpromazine 50 mg IM or hyoscine 0·5 mg IM. Routine treatment should be started with prochlorperazine 10 mg three times a day or promethazine 25 mg three times a day.

Intractable symptoms justify a surgical destruction of the labyrinth. Between attacks, caloric tests are of little help in making the diagnosis.

Vestibular neuronitis (acute labyrinthitis)

This condition often occurs in small epidemics and consists of acute vertigo, accompanied by nystagmus, nausea, vomiting and prostration. The attack begins to subside within a few days and the patient is quite well again at the end of two weeks. The site of the lesion is unknown but may be intracranial as there is sometimes a mild, lymphocytic reaction in the cerebrospinal fluid. After an attack the response to caloric stimulation is sometimes lost on the affected side, but it may also remain normal. Hearing is unaffected.

An acute vestibular upset may complicate the use of *streptomycin*. It is unusual for any toxic effects to result from a short course, but the possibility should be borne in mind when it is used for long periods. When streptomycin is used in the treatment of urinary tract infections the likelihood is increased as the ability to excrete the streptomycin may be impaired.

Acute vertigo may result from a brain-stem plaque in *disseminated sclerosis*. The symptoms usually persist for a week or two but sometimes for several months.

Chapter 23
The Differential Diagnosis of Disease of the Spinal Cord

1. Compression of the spinal cord:
    A. tumour;
    B. cervical spondylosis.
2. Subacute combined degeneration of the cord.

The Differential Diagnosis of Disease of the Spinal Cord

3. Motor neuron disease.
4. Syringomyelia.
5. Meningovascular syphilis.
6. Disseminated sclerosis.
7. Transverse myelitis.
8. Hereditary ataxia.

From the history and examination one should determine:

(a) the age of the patient at the onset of the disease; the rate at which the disease has developed; any evidence of remission.

(b) the site of the lesion; any evidence of selective system involvement.

(c) the extent of the lesion; how many segments are involved; is it the result of one or several scattered lesions?

Ancillary investigations may include:

(d) straight X-rays of the spine.

(e) lumbar puncture with particular attention to the dynamics and constituents of the cerebrospinal fluid.

(f) myelography.

(g) examination of the blood: estimation of vitamin B12 levels, FTA.

(1) Compression of the spinal cord

A. **Tumour** (p. 156)

(a) Any age: variable rate of progression. No remission. Pain is often present.

(b) Transverse cord lesion: no selective system involvement.

(c) Usually extends over one or two segments.

(e) CSF: partial or complete block on manometry. Protein raised with extramedullary tumour.

(f) Myelogram demonstrates presence of tumour.

B. **Cervical spondylosis** (p. 158)

(a) Middle aged and elderly. Gradually progressive. Often intermittent at first, but no true remission. Pain a prominent feature.

(b) Transverse cord lesion and nerve root involvement in the cervical region.

(d) Spondylotic changes on X-ray.

(e) CSF: partial or complete block. Protein normal or slightly raised.
(f) Myelography: evidence of disc protrusion.

(2) Subacute combined degeneration of the cord (p. 162)

(a) Middle aged and elderly. Gradually progressive. Remissions uncommon.
(b) Pyramidal tracts and posterior columns especially affected. Also peripheral neuropathy.
(g) Macrocytic anaemia. Megaloblastic marrow. Serum vitamin B12 less than 50 $\mu\mu$ gm per ml.

(3) Motor neuron disease (p. 165)

(a) Middle aged: variable rate of progression. No remission.
(b) The motor system is exclusively affected: both upper and lower motor neurons.
(c) Involvement may extend to the motor nuclei of the brain-stem.

(4) Syringomyelia (p. 169)

(a) Below the age of thirty years. Very slowly progressive. Periods of arrest but no true remission.
(b) Most commonly in the cervical region: selective loss of pain and temperature sensation at the level of the lesion.
(c) Lesions extends over several segments, often into the lower brain-stem.
(d) X-rays: widening of the spinal canal.
(f) Myelography may show expansion of the cord.

(5) Meningovascular syphilis (p. 113)

(a) Middle aged: variably progressive, often with a step-like deterioration, and partial remissions.
(c) There is usually some involvement of the cranial nerves: Argyll-Robertson pupils.
(e) CSF: lymphocytosis. Protein content increased; mid-zone gold curve. WR usually positive.
(g) Blood FTA positive.

(6) Disseminated sclerosis (p. 172)

(a) Most commonly in youth and middle age, occasionally in late middle age. Variable progression, usually with clear-cut remissions and relapses.

(c) Scattered lesions throughout the CNS. There is usually some evidence of intracranial involvement, and eye signs are common.

(e) CSF. In half the cases some abnormality is found. Lymphocytosis, moderate rise in protein content, first or mid-zone gold curve. FTA negative. Oligoclonal bands.

(7) Transverse myelitis (p. 177)

(a) Youth and middle age: subacute onset. Remission after several weeks.

(b) Transverse cord lesion.

(c) Two or three segments affected. There is also a progessive form involving several segments. There may be an accompanying optic neuritis.

(e) CSF. Manometry normal. Slight rise in cells and protein. FTA negative.

(f) Myelography normal.

(8) Hereditary ataxias (p. 179)

(a) Usually before the age of thirty years. Very slowly progressive. No remission. Family history.

(b) Combination of spasticity and cerebellar ataxia. There are commonly bony stigmata such as pes cavus and scoliosis.

(e) CSF normal. FTA negative.

Chapter 24
Compression of the Spinal Cord

Compression of the spinal cord can result from:
(1) **Tumours of the spinal cord:**
   (a) Intramedullary (within the substance of the cord).
   (b) Extramedullary (outside the spinal cord).

(2) **Extradural lesions,** e.g., abscess, leukaemic deposits.

(3) **Diseases of the vertebral column**
   (a) Cervical spondylosis (p. 158).
   (b) Fracture dislocation of the spine.
   (c) Tumours of the vertebral bodies.
   (d) Osteitis deformans (Paget's disease of the bone).
   (e) Tuberculosis of the vertebral bodies (Pott's disease).

Compression of the spinal cord results in paraplegia, which may be spastic or flaccid (p. 54). It constitutes a surgical emergency. Once the diagnosis is made, the patient should be referred to a neurosurgeon. Direct pressure may cause necrosis of the cord which is irreversible. Damage may also result from ischaemia caused by compression of the spinal arteries or from congestion secondary to venous occlusion. The prompt relief of cord compression is followed by a reversal of dysfunction which is secondary to vascular changes.

TUMOURS OF THE SPINAL CORD

Intramedullary tumours are uncommon. They develop from the glial or ependymal cells of the cord and correspond histologically with the various types of cerebral tumours (p. 102). The rate at which signs develop varies according to the malignancy of the tumour, but in general it is more rapid than in a histologically similar cerebral tumour. This is due to the smaller volume of the spinal canal and the crowding of structures in the cord. The signs are less well defined than in extramedullary lesions and the tumour usually extends over several segments of the cord.

Pain is seldom an outstanding symptom, but dissociated sensory loss and unpleasant sensations of coldness are common. Sphincter dysfunction occurs earlier with intramedullary tumours than with those arising outside the cord.

The changes in the cerebrospinal fluid are often insignificant. Myelography and surgical exploration are necessary before the diagnosis is complete.

Extramedullary tumours are more common. They develop outside the substance of the spinal cord. They grow slowly and compress rather than invade the neural tissue. Meningiomas occur in the dorsal region and neurofibromas are more often found in the cervical region.

The earliest symptoms are due to involvement of the nerve roots. Pain is a prominent feature. It often precedes other symptoms by weeks or months. Paraesthesiae and numbness develop in the dermatome of the affected nerve root and a symptomatic herpes sometimes erupts in the same distribution. It has been suggested that the mechanical irritation activates a previously dormant virus. The majority of extramedullary tumours are situated on the postero-lateral convexity of the cord and so the sensory symptoms are more marked than the lower motor neuron signs.

The increasing size of the tumour causes unilateral compression of the cord with the development of a *Brown-Séquard syndrome* (p. 55). This is often incomplete or on the other hand the compression may involve both halves of the cord giving rise to paraplegia (p. 54). The sphincters are rarely affected in the early months of the disease.

Changes in the cerebrospinal fluid occur early. There is a great increase in the protein content (up to 30 g/l) and the fluid may clot in the tube (Froin's syndrome). The dynamics of the fluid are altered. The Queckenstedt manoeuvre may disclose a complete block or a sluggish rise and fall in the pressure. If the symptoms and signs suggest a diagnosis of spinal cord tumour, a lumbar puncture should not be performed unless there is ready access to a neurosurgical department. The removal of a few millilitres of cerebrospinal fluid may be sufficient to cause a displacement of the tumour and so precipitate irreversible cord damage.

Intraspinal neurofibromata sometimes occur as part of a generalized neurofibromatosis (*von Recklinghausen's disease*). This consists of subcutaneous nodules on the peripheral nerves; diffuse fibromata on the nerve trunks, accompanied by overgrowths of skin (plexiform neuromata); multiple pedunculated and sessile skin tumours; pigmented areas on the skin; and bony changes, the most common of which is kyphoscoliosis.

Treatment
The surgical removal of benign extramedullary tumours is highly successful. If the diagnosis and treatment are delayed, the compression may result in irreversible damage to the cord. A well-defined intramedullary tumour may occasionally be resectable, but more often a decompressive laminectomy and radiotherapy is given.

CERVICAL SPONDYLOSIS

This is a disease of the spinal cord and nerve roots, secondary to degenerative changes in the cervical vertebrae (Fig. 28).

Aetiology

The intervertebral disc is composed of two structurally different parts; a gelatinous central nucleus pulposus which is surrounded by a tough annulus fibrosus. With advancing age there is a gradual dessication of the nucleus, and it consequently shrinks. This throws unusual stresses on the annulus, causing bony outgrowths to develop at the points of its ligamentous attachment to the adjacent vertebrae. These are called osteophytes. Part of the annulus may bulge posteriorly into the spinal canal, or laterally into the intervertebral foramina. Encroachment upon the intervertebral foramina either by a bulging annulus or by osteophytes results in an inflammatory reaction in the dural nerve root sleeves, compression of the nerve root and interference with the segmental blood supply. Posterior protrusion of the annulus fibrosus may compress the spinal cord directly or occlude the anterior spinal artery. This can cause ischaemia in the adjacent spinal segments so that the neurological signs are more extensive than would be suggested by the discs directly involved.

Evidence of disc degeneration and the other changes may be obtained by X-ray examination of the cervical spine. Antero-posterior, lateral and oblique views should be taken. Narrowing of

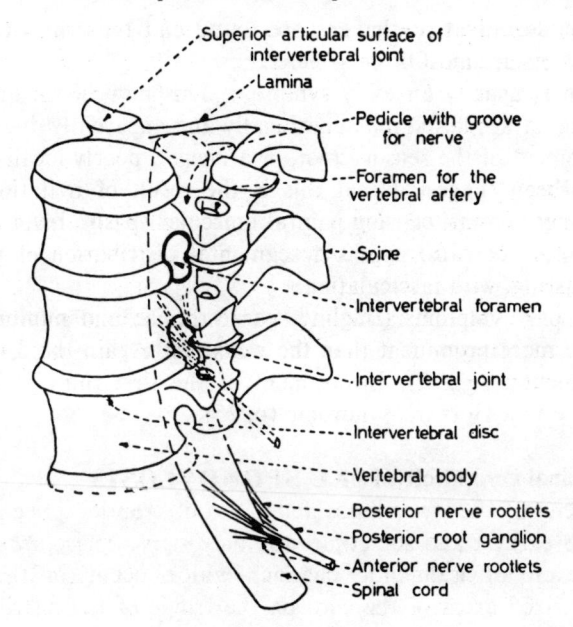

Fig. 28. Oblique view of the mid cervical spine.

the disc spaces, osteophyte formation and encroachment on the intervertebral foramina may be seen. These X-ray abnormalities are found in 60 per cent of the population over the age of fifty years, and so may be considered to be part of the normal ageing process.

Although cervical spondylosis is a common disease, only a small proportion of the population with radiological changes actually present with neurological signs. Repeated minor injuries, contortion of the neck, or even a congenitally narrow spinal canal may be responsible for the variable morbidity.

There are three groups of *symptoms:*
1. Those due to compression of the nerve roots.
2. Those due to involvement of the spinal cord.
3. Those due to local disease in the cervical spine.

Most commonly the patient presents with a combination of all three symptomatologies.

(1) Compression of the nerve roots
The greater part of cervical flexion and extension occurs at the C5–6 and C6–7 intervertebral discs. Consequently this is where the

bulk of degenerative changes are found and thus the C6 and C7 nerve roots are most often affected.

Pain is usually an early symptom. This may be an unpleasant burning paraesthesia, felt superficially and apparently due to direct involvement of the sensory root, or a deeper, poorly localized ache. It has been suggested that this is the result of irritation of the motor nerve roots, causing painful muscular spasm. Involvement of the motor root also causes a segmental distribution of weakness and wasting, with fasciculation.

Sensory symptoms (tingling, paraesthesiae and numbness) are usually more prominent than the weakness. Again the distribution is segmental (Fig. 7). Involvement of the first thoracic root will give rise to a Horner's syndrome (p. 25).

(2) Spinal cord involvement

Spasticity of the lower limbs and a loss of proprioceptive sensation are the earliest and sometimes the only signs. These are probably the result of ischaemic changes which occur in the poorly vascularized areas of the cord on the fringe of the distribution of the main (sulcal) branch of the anterior spinal artery and the penetrating branches of the coronal artery (p. 54). Later a spastic paraplegia with interruption of all forms of sensation below the lesion may develop due to direct compression of the cord. Such a complete transection is uncommon and suggests the subluxation of one vertebral body on another.

(3) Local disease in the cervical spine

If questioned, the patient will often describe an ill-localized ache or stiffness in the neck, but these symptoms rarely dominate the clinical picture. Examination of neck movements usually reveals some limitation particularly on extension or lateral flexion, although this is by no means universal. The limitation of movement may be accompanied by pain which is felt across the shoulders. Cervical spondylosis is sometimes responsible for a suboccipital headache. This results from spasm of the cervical muscles, which is caused by mechanical irritation of the motor nerve roots.

Diagnosis

The disease usually develops in late middle age, with signs of an advancing spastic paraparesis and wasting, weakness and sometimes fasciculation in the upper limbs. This can easily be confused with motor neuron disease. It is important to diagnose cervical spondylosis correctly as this condition is potentially remediable. The diagnosis is not made any easier by the fact that the majority of patients with motor neuron disease, subacute combined degeneration of the cord, syringomyelia and disseminated sclerosis in the appropriate age group have the X-ray changes of cervical spondylosis.

Nerve root lesions must be distinguished from Pancoast's syndrome, the thoracic inlet syndrome, injuries to the brachial plexus (see below) and neuralgic amyotrophy.

Straight X-rays of the cervical spine will suggest the diagnosis but if surgical relief is contemplated, myelography will be required. Myodil, a radiopaque oil, is introduced by lumbar puncture after the withdrawal of CSF for examination. By the appropriate positioning of the patients, radiographs will demonstrate any encroachment on the spinal canal or nerve roots.

The CSF often shows a slight (0.5–0.8 gl^{-1}) rise in the protein content.

Treatment
In the mild cases or where there has been an acute onset of nerve root symptoms, conservative treatment is indicated. Neck traction often relieves the pain and this should be followed by exercises to strengthen the axial muscles which maintain the stability of the cervical spine. An immobilizing collar will usually relieve the root symptoms but there is a likelihood of relapse when the collar is discarded.

Evidence of cord compression or progressive disability is an indication for surgical treatment. This is directed to the relief of local compression by osteophytes or the extruded disc. Symptoms of nerve root involvement can often be relieved, and the advance of the disease checked. It is unlikely that established signs of cord involvement can be reversed.

Injuries to the nerve roots may occur in motor accidents but are most often seen following obstetrical injuries. The 5th and 6th cervical roots are sometimes damaged during birth by downward traction on the shoulder. This results in weakness of the deltoids, biceps, brachioradialis and the supinators of the wrists—*Erb's palsy*. The arm hangs at the patient's side, internally rotated (the policeman's tip position). If the arm is splinted in abduction at the shoulder the prognosis is good.

Injury to the first thoracic root results from abduction injuries at the shoulder. There is weakness and wasting of the small muscles of the hand (*Klumpke's paralysis*). The prognosis for recovery of power is poor.

Pancoast's superior sulcus tumour of the lung commonly invades the lower cervical and upper thoracic nerve roots causing severe pain in the arm, segmental weakness and sensory loss, and a Horner's syndrome. A chest X-ray is diagnostic.

Thoracic inlet syndrome
This condition most often affects middle-aged women. It is usually precipitated by muscular hypotonia allowing the shoulder girdle to droop. This puts an unusual tension on the lower trunk of the brachial plexus where it is angled over the first rib. The angulation may be exaggerated by the presence of a cervical rib or a fibrous band which sometimes extends from the seventh cervical vertebra to the first rib. Pain is the most prominent symptom, but it is often accompanied by numbness along the medial border of the hand and wasting of the small muscles of the hand. The pain is worsened by carrying heavy weights or even wearing a heavy overcoat.

Symptomatic relief is obtained by exercises to strengthen the muscles of the shoulder girdle. The persistence of symptoms in spite of conservative treatment is an indication for the resection of a cervical rib.

Chapter 25
Subacute Combined Degeneration of the Cord

In spite of the restriction that its name implies, this disease affects the brain and the peripheral nerves in addition to the spinal cord.

Subacute Combined Degeneration of the Cord

The brunt of the damage in the cord falls on the pyramidal tracts and the posterior columns. The patient most often presents with peripheral paraesthesiae and spastic ataxia, accompanying a megaloblastic anaemia.

Aetiology

Subacute combined degeneration of the cord results from a deficiency of cyanocobalamin (vitamin B12). The serum level of vitamin B12 in this disorder is less than 50 pg ml^{-1}. Normal diets contain ample quantities of vitamin B12, but the presence of a transport factor, the 'intrinsic factor' is necessary for its absorption from the small bowel. The intrinsic factor is secreted in association with hydrochloric acid by the mucosa of the stomach. Gastric mucosal atrophy and an achlorhydria which fails to respond to maximal doses (0·04 mg per kg bodyweight) of histamine is the most common cause of vitamin B12 deficiency.

A deficiency of vitamin B12 impairs the maturation of the red blood cells giving rise to a megaloblastic anaemia. This usually precedes the development of neurological signs, but occasionally the peripheral blood picture remains normal in spite of a total absence of circulating vitamin B12. The practice of using 'blood tonics' which contain small quantities of vitamin B12 has sometimes suppressed the development of anaemia while allowing the neurological signs to develop unchecked. The folic acid content of such preparations may precipitate neurological disease.

Pathology
The chief pathological feature is a destruction of myelin. This occurs in small patches which eventually coalesce. The demyelination is most apparent in the posterior columns and the pyramidal tracts of the spinal cord, but in severe cases scarcely any of the white matter of the cord or brain escapes. Degeneration of the nerve fibres which traverse the affected areas follows rapidly on the initial demyelination. The peripheral nerves also show evidence of degeneration but the nerve cell bodies are seldom affected.

Clinical features
The disease affects both men and women and usually develops in late middle age. Almost without exception, the first symptom is of tingling and numbness affecting the toes and later the fingers. This

spreads proximally in the typical glove and stocking distribution. There may be no objective signs for several weeks but cutaneous hypaesthesia eventually develops in the same areas. It may be accompanied by tenderness of the calf muscles. The upper level of the sensory disturbance is often marked by a feeling of irritating tightness.

An early sign of cord involvement is a profound loss of proprioception The patient feels that the ground is insecure beneath his feet and he stands and walks on a wide base. He is more unsteady when his eyes are closed (Rombergism), and on clinical examination it is found that his sense of vibration is diminished or absent. Soon after this he develops spastic weakness of his legs. The knee jerks are increased although the ankle jerks are frequently diminished or absent due to the earlier involvement of the peripheral nerves. The plantar responses are almost always extensor. Severe spasticity may give rise to flexor withdrawal spasms of the legs. Involvement of the sphincters is delayed until the other signs of cord damage are well established. Hesitancy, urgency and, less often, retention occur.

The optic nerves are not uncommonly affected by the pathological process. There may be a frank optic atrophy or sometimes an earlier sign of involvement is the development of bilateral central scotomata and constriction of the visual fields. The pupils are often small but react normally.

The deficiency of vitamin B12 has a direct effect on the metabolism of the brain cells. This not uncommonly results in symptoms of mental disorder consisting of disorientation, apathy and mild dementia.

The constituents of the cerebrospinal fluid are normal and the FTA is negative.

The patient is usually pale and his tongue is characteristically smooth and red. He may complain of breathlessness and of being readily fatigued. The anaemia is often severe with a hyperactive bone marrow showing evidence of megaloblastic changes.

Diagnosis
The fully developed neurological picture accompanied by a megaloblastic anaemia presents no diagnostic difficulty. Not uncommonly the peripheral blood is normal but there is almost without exception an absolute achlorhydria. In rare instances the

patient may present with dementia. Spontaneous remissions occasionally occur.

The level of serum vitamin B12 is less than 50 pg ml^{-1}, and the absorption of cyanocobalamin labelled with radioactive cobalt is diminished (Schilling test).

The diagnosis should be considered in every case of progressive cord disease as the results of delayed diagnosis are so serious and the effect of early treatment is so good.

Treatment

Hydroxocobalamin, 1000 μg, by intramuscular injection daily for 3 days and then fortnightly. This treatment must be continued for the duration of the patient's life.

There is an early recovery from any mental symptoms. Peripheral neuropathy can be expected to recover, and improvement continues over a period of 4–6 months. There is usually a lessening of the symptoms and signs due to cord damage, but the recovery is seldom complete. The patient will require physiotherapy, and especially co-ordination exercises to help him overcome the ataxia.

The severely anaemic patient should be nursed in bed until the haemoglobin rises to 7 g per 100 ml and he will require iron supplements.

Chapter 26
Motor Neuron Disease

This is a progressive disease whose clinical manifestations affect the motor system exclusively. Both the upper and lower motor neurons are involved. Either may dominate the clinical picture, but more often the signs are of a combined lesion.

Aetiology

An apparently identical disease which affects a closely inbred native group in the Mariana Islands is inherited. The inherited factor is probably a metabolic abnormality of the motor neuron. The familial occurrence of motor neuron disease is, however, rare in other countries. Pathologically it is a chronic degenerative process which primarily affects the anterior horn cells of the spinal cord, the motor nuclei in the brain-stem and the corticospinal fibres. The motor cells in the cerebral cortex are affected later and less severely. An association is sometimes suggested between injury, lead poisoning or previous acute anterior poliomyelitis, and the eventual development of motor neuron disease. It is possible that these factors may hasten the appearance of the disease, but no good evidence of a causal relationship exists.

It affects men more frequently than women and usually develops in late middle age.

A combined presentation of upper and lower motor neuron signs is called amyotrophic lateral sclerosis. Progressive muscular atrophy is the name given to the disease when only lower neuron signs are present. If the disease initially affects the motor nuclei of the medulla it is called progressive bulbar palsy. Primary lateral sclerosis is an uncommon variety, consisting solely of upper motor neuron signs.

Amyotrophic lateral sclerosis
The onset of symptoms is characteristically insidious. Fatigue and muscle pain often precede the appearance of weakness and wasting. Sometimes it is the wasting which first draws the disease to the patient's notice. The interossei and the muscles of the thenar eminence are affected early. The two hands are often unequally involved and the early signs may seem to have a segmental distribution. The wasting and weakness usually spread proximally to involve the muscles of the shoulder girdle and the trunk, but may occasionally start there and spread distally. Fasciculation (p. 9) is a prominent sign. It is often most obvious in the first dorsal interosseus, the deltoid and the pectoralis muscles. It is most apparent when the patient relaxes after vigorous muscular effort, or when the muscle is percussed with a tendon hammer.

Upper motor neuron signs in the lower limbs accompany the weakness, wasting and fasciculation in the arms. There is usually a spastic weakness of the legs with increased tendon jerks and extensor plantar responses. Upper motor neuron signs may also extend to the upper limbs so that there is a paradoxical increase in the reflexes accompanying the wasting and fasciculation.

As the disease advances fasciculation and other signs of lower motor neuron involvement appear in the lower limbs. Eventually the muscles innervated by the motor nuclei of the medulla are affected, giving rise to a bulbar palsy (see below). Aspiration pneumonia is the most frequent cause of death. This occurs within 4–5 years of the onset of the disease in the majority of cases; the process occasionally becomes static and some patients live for 8–10 years after the diagnosis is made.

Progressive muscular atrophy
In progressive muscular atrophy, the signs of disease are limited to a lower motor neuron disorder, which often remains localized for several years. The duration of life is usually longer than in the case of amyotrophic lateral sclerosis. Apart from the absence of upper motor neuron signs this form of the disease is identical with amyotrophic lateral sclerosis. Histological examination of the cord shows that the pyramidal tracts are involved in spite of the absence of clinical signs.

Progressive bulbar palsy
Involvement of the motor nuclei of the brain-stem affects:
  the muscles of the tongue (hypoglossal nuclei);
  the muscles of mastication (trigeminal motor nuclei);
  the muscles of deglutition (glossopharyngeal and vagal nuclei);
  the facial muscles (facial nuclei).
  At first the patient finds it difficult to protrude his tongue fully, and the weakness can be assessed by asking him to push his tongue into his cheek. He may find that when he lies flat, his tongue falls back against the soft palate making him choke. Later the tongue lies immobile, atrophied and fibrillating. The circumoral muscles are affected early, making it difficult for the patient to close his lips. Saliva dribbles from his mouth and the combined weaknesses of lips and tongue give rise to dysarthria. Palatal weakness allows fluids to regurgitate down the nose and finally the patient is unable to swallow or close his jaw.
  The extra-ocular muscles are not affected.
  The development of bulbar palsy usually results in the death of the patient within a year or two, due to aspiration pneumonia.
  The 'bulbar muscles' may be involved in an upper motor neuron paralysis. In this case, the distribution of the muscles affected is the same, but it is a spastic rather than a flaccid weakness. The

most striking difference is in the appearance of the tongue, which is small and stiff, instead of soft and fibrillating. The jaw jerk in this 'pseudo-bulbar palsy' is brisk.

Diagnosis
It is essential that any treatable condition should be distinguished from motor neuron disease. Unless lower motor neuron signs are found in the lower limbs, cervical spondylosis and spinal cord tumour can mimic amyotrophic lateral sclerosis so closely that a myelogram may be necessary for their recognition. In motor neuron disease the myelogram and the constituents of the cerebrospinal fluid are normal. Syringomyelia and subacute combined degeneration of the cord both present with prominent sensory symptoms. The progressive spinal form of disseminated sclerosis may be indistinguishable from primary lateral sclerosis unless there are cranial nerve signs or abnormal constituents in the cerebrospinal fluid.

Treatment
At present there is no curative treatment for this disease. If muscle cramps are distressing, they can be alleviated with procaine amide 0·25 g four times a day. In cases of bulbar paralysis soft porridgy food is most easily swallowed, but nasogastric feeds eventually become necessary.

Kugelberg-Welander syndrome: a hereditary, proximal spinal muscular atrophy. This condition is similar to motor neuron disease, but occurs from the first year of life to adolescence. It affects the proximal limb muscles and fasciculation is seen. There is a non-sex-linked recessive inheritance. Progression of the illness is slow. It may be confused with limb-girdle muscular dystrophy, but can be distinguished by biopsy or electromyography.

Chapter 27
Syringomyelia

This is a disease which most often affects the cervical region of the spinal cord and is characterized by dissociated sensory loss, lower motor neuron weakness and trophic changes in the upper limbs, and spasticity of the legs.

Aetiology
Syringomyelia is often associated with such congenital anomalies as spina bifida and naevi over the spine. This suggests that it is a result of imperfect fusion of the neural tube.

In other cases, it has been shown that the cavity in the spinal cord (the syrinx) is continuous with the fourth ventricle. This is likely to occur if the foramen of Magendie is partially occluded so that the pulse wave of cerebrospinal fluid is funnelled into the upper part of the central canal of the spinal cord. The wall of the canal may then rupture permitting fistulous tracks to develop in the tissue of the cord. Distortion of the medullary architecture, occluding the foramen of Magendie, is commonly a consequence of the Arnold-Chiari malformation (a downward displacement of the medulla and cerebellum through the foramen magnum).

The cavitation extends over several segments from the upper cervical region to the upper thoracic. Due to the central position of the cavity those fibres which cross the mid-line of the cord in the anterior commissure are particularly affected by the pathological process. There is thus a loss of pain and temperature sensation in the dermatomes of both sides of the body related to the affected segments of the cord. Light touch sensation and proprioception travelling in the ipsilateral posterior columns are unaffected. Thus, the sensory loss is 'dissociated'.

The anterior horn cells are affected in about half the cases giving rise to typical lower neuron wasting and weakness. Pressure on the pyramidal tracts causes a spastic paraparesis. Trophic changes in the hands result from involvement of the descending sympathetic pathways in the cervical cord and the sympathetic cell bodies in the upper thoracic segments. A Horner's syndrome (p. 25) is commonly found.

There is sometimes a continuous cavity from the cervical cord up into the medulla. Cavitation may also occur in the brain stem as an isolated finding (syringobulbia). In the medulla the cavity is situated dorsolaterally so that the neurological signs are usually asymmetrical. The decussating fibres from the spinal nucleus of the trigeminal nerve, the 'bulbar' motor nuclei (cranial nerves IX, X, XI, XII) and the connections of the vestibular nuclei are characteristically involved.

A prolapse of the cerebellar tonsils through the foramen magnum compresses the lower medulla, mimicking the clinical features of syringobulbia.

Clinical features
The development of symptoms is usually insidious, but some patients describe the acute onset of pain in the neck and arm as a consequence of violent physical effort.

There is loss of pain and temperature sensation which typically affects the upper limbs and the upper three or four thoracic dermatomes on the trunk. Dull aches and intense stabbing pains are sometimes felt in these areas. The patient frequently suffers painless burns on the hands, which due to the analgesia are often neglected. This results in them becoming infected, which in addition to the trophic changes makes them slow to heal. The skin becomes hairless and thickened, particularly over the hands, so that the fingers look like a bunch of bananas.

Repeated painless injuries to the joints give rise to changes which are comparable with those seen in tabes—Charcot joints. The elbows are most often affected.

The lower motor neuron signs are frequently asymmetrical so that one hand is much more severely affected than the other. The small muscles of the hand, which are innervated by the lower cervical and upper thoracic segments, become weak and atrophied. The flexors of the fingers are often spared so that a claw hand develops. The tendon reflexes are diminished in the affected segments.

Examination of the legs reveals mild bilateral spasticity with brisk reflexes and extensor plantar responses. The patient may feel that his legs are stiff and easily fatigued but complaints of weakness are infrequent. Sphincter disturbances are uncommon.

Syringobulbia is almost invariably accompanied by nystagmus. A lower medullary or upper cervical lesion interrupts the decussating fibres from the spinal nucleus of the trigeminal nerve causing a loss of pain sensation in a strip in front of the ear and along the jaw (p. 39). The main sensory nucleus of the trigeminal nerve is involved if the cavity extends higher in the medulla causing a complete hemifacial anaesthesia. The medial lemniscus may be affected with a resulting contralateral loss of proprioception and light touch sensation. An asymmetrical lower motor neuron lesion of the tongue, palate and laryngeal muscles is commonly seen.

Diagnosis
An intramedullary cord tumour or uncommonly haemorrhage into the substance of the cord (haematomyelia) may give rise to symptoms and signs which are indistinguishable from syringomyelia. The development of signs due to tumour or haematomyelia is generally more acute and rapidly progressive than in the case of syringomyelia.

The distinctive sensory loss makes it possible to separate syringomyelia from those other conditions which cause wasting of the small muscles of the hands, motor neuron disease, cervical spondylosis and peripheral nerve lesions.

X-ray examination of the cervical spine may show widening of the spinal canal and X-rays of the cervico-occipital junction may show basilar impression. Myodil myelography displays the swollen cord which collapses during gas myelography.

Treatment
With the recognition of a syrinx which communicates with the ventricular system there is a prospect of treating this condition surgically. Decompression of the posterior fossa with the dissection of the foramen of Magendie may re-establish the normal flow of CSF, prevent further expansion of the syrinx and possibly promote some resolution of the existing symptoms.

Chapter 28
The Demyelinating Diseases

The common feature of this group of diseases is that the primary pathological change is demyelination of the nerve fibres in the central nervous system.

Disseminated sclerosis, transverse myelitis, neuromyelitis optica and acute discholomyelitis will be described in this chapter. Primary demyelination also occurs in subacute combined degeneration of the cord (p. 162).

There is good evidence that acute disseminated encephalomyelitis results from an allergic response in the tissue of the nervous system initiated by a preceding infection. The enigma of disseminated sclerosis remains unsolved. Epidemiological studies suggest that it would be compatible with the response of an individual who has inherited immune deficiencies and has been exposed to a neuropathic enterovirus in childhood or adolescence.

DISSEMINATED SCLEROSIS

This is one of the common neurological disorders affecting young people. Its characteristic course consists of a series of apparently isolated attacks affecting different parts of the central nervous system. Each attack subsequently shows some degree of remission, but the overall picture is one of deterioration.

Pathology

Each separate clinical attack is caused by an episode of demyelination in the cerebrospinal axis. At post-mortem the lesions are most prominent in the pyramidal tracts and the posterior columns of the cord, around the ventricles of the brain, in the optic nerves, and in the pons and medulla, especially involving the cerebellar peduncles.

In the acute phase, the affected area is oedematous, and infiltrated with lymphocytes and plasma cells. This infiltration is most apparent round the veins, but the area of demyelination itself is not directly related to the position of blood vessels. Scavenger cells remove the globules of degenerating myelin and as the acute phase subsides there is a reactive gliosis. The end result is a shrunken area of sclerosis. The axis cylinders and the nerve cell bodies are not directly affected.

The symptoms which are due to demyelination are irreversible, but as the oedema in the surrounding tissue is reabsorbed there is a substantial return of function which may obscure the underlying deficit. Each attack develops over a period of a few days, and then begins to remit after a further 2–6 weeks. The remission can be remarkably complete so that no abnormality is found on examination, but more often some slight stigma remains. A relapse is often associated with such events as colds and chills, injuries, extremes of fatigue and exposure to inclement weather.

The illness is more common in temperate climates and is virtually unknown in the tropics. It most commonly presents in young people, from the age of 20 to 45 years. Less often, the first identifiable symptom appears in the sixth or seventh decade. Earlier symptoms may have been unrecognized or forgotten and at post-mortem the lesions are usually more numerous and extensive than the clinical picture would have suggested.

Clinical features
The clinical diagnosis depends upon the demonstration of physical signs which can only be explained by lesions in at least two sites in the central nervous system.

The first episode of demyelination may occur at any site in the white matter of the brain or spinal cord. Most often the early lesions affect either the pyramidal tract, causing tiredness and dragging of one leg, or the optic nerve resulting in impaired vision and pain in the eye. If the illness develops in middle age it may present as a gradually progressive spastic paraplegia, clinically difficult to distinguish from cord compression.

Any combination of symptoms and signs may coexist.

Spastic weakness of the limbs. Tiredness and heaviness in one leg is a common presenting symptom. The patient scuffs the toe of his shoe, tending to trip on rough ground. Spasticity may be accompanied by a dull ache in the leg and there is frequently a complaint that the legs jump spontaneously, particularly when the patient is in bed. More profound spasticity is accompanied by painful spasm of the muscles, which results in exaggerated withdrawal responses of the lower limbs. Extensor spasm may occur, but is less common. The tendon reflexes are brisk, often with clonus at the knees and ankles, the abdominal reflexes are diminished or absent, and the plantar response is extensor.

Not uncommonly the symptoms are restricted to one leg while signs are found bilaterally. An increase in the tendon jerks of one or both arms is common, but weakness is usually less prominent. The jaw jerk may be increased.

Bladder. Lesions in the corticospinal tracts often cause disorders of sphincter control. Hesitancy, urgency and frequency are common. Acute retention and incontinence of urine also occur. Impotence is not unusual.

Sensory disorders. Paraesthesiae and dysaesthesiae are often prominent, while complete anaesthesia is uncommon. Proprioceptive disorders occur frequently giving rise to a sensory ataxia and inco-ordination of the arms. Vibration sense is usually diminished at the ankles.

If there is a lesion in the posterior columns of the cervical cord, flexion of the neck causes tingling, shock-like sensations to run down the arms to the fingers or down the legs (Lhermitte's sign).

Distinct sensory levels are sometimes found on the trunk simulating a compressive cord lesion. There is often a sensation of tightness at the upper level of the sensory loss. An area of demyelination in the brain-stem occasionally gives rise to a symptomatic form of trigeminal neuralgia. Unlike idiopathic trigeminal neuralgia it may be accompanied by hypaesthesia over the affected side of the face.

Retrobulbar neuritis. The patient develops increasingly blurred vision in one eye, which may progress to complete uniocular blindness during a period of a few hours or two to three days. The affected eye is often painful, particularly when the patient looks to the side. The eyeball may feel tender when touched. If the site of demyelination is immediately behind the optic nerve head, the disc will be pink and swollen. Otherwise the appearance of the fundus is quite normal. If the visual loss is not complete, a central scotoma can usually be detected on confrontation. This may only be apparent if a coloured objective is used.

As the symptoms subside over the next few weeks, the size of the scotoma diminishes and atrophic changes may be seen in the temporal half of the optic disc. Dark radiating streaks from the optic disc are thought to be due to demyelination of the nerve fibres in the retina.

Retrobulbar neuritis also occurs as an isolated lesion, with no evidence of generalized involvement of the nervous system. There may be recurrent attacks affecting the same eye.

Asymptomatic optic neuritis may be detected by delayed visual evoked responses (VERs).

Diplopia is a common symptom, but it is less usual to find any objective paralysis of the ocular muscles.

Cerebellar signs. The lesions are most commonly found in the cerebellar peduncles rather than in the cerebellum itself.

Nystagmus: a coarse, horizontal nystagmus which is made more prominent by lateral deviation of the eyes. Vertical nystagmus, or nystagmus which is limited to the abducting eye are firm evidence of a brain-stem lesion.

Dyssynergia: a fragmentation of voluntary movements resulting in intention tremor, dysdiadochokinesis and incoordination in the heel–shin test. Ataxic gait and disorders of postural control, accompanied by muscular hypotonia.

Titubation: a continuous, rhythmical tremor of the head and trunk. This may be so severe as to prevent the patient from standing unaided, and make dressing and feeding almost impossible.

Dysarthria is common.

Disorders of mood. Euphoria: an unrealistic feeling of well-being affects about a third of all patients.

Depression can also occur.

Cerebrospinal fluid
The constituents of the cerebrospinal fluid are abnormal in half of the cases. The protein is raised but amounts in excess of 1 g l^{-1} are uncommon. The gamma globulin fraction is commonly increased (IgG>12 per cent). Electrophoresis of the CSF often shows that the normally unitary gammaglobulin fraction is broken into a number of narrow bands—the oligoclonal bands. There is sometimes a lymphocytosis during a relapse and a first or second zone gold curve may be found.

Prognosis

The progression of disseminated sclerosis is extremely variable. There are, however, four distinctive clinical presentations.

1. The classical picture of intermittent relapses, followed by more or less complete remissions. With each ensuing attack the remissions are usually less complete, so that within 10–20 years the patient is physically disabled.
2. A rapid deterioration with numerous relapses and only partial remission occurring in the first year or two of the illness. Within this period the patient is often severely incapacitated.
3. Infrequent attacks with long periods of remission.
4. Continuous deterioration without remission.

The particular clinical variety can usually be determined within 2–3 years of the appearance of the first symptom. With a few exceptions the disease will then continue to develop along its declared path.

In general, new lesions appear within the first 7 or 8 years of the illness. Thereafter, further deterioration is more gradual and often the result of decreasing physical activity.

Diagnosis

The diagnosis is usually made on a clear history of relapses and remissions and signs of multiple lesions in the central nervous system. In the progressive spinal form of disseminated sclerosis, both the symptoms and signs may resemble those of cord compression so closely that myelography is necessary to distinguish between them. If there are eye signs, delayed VERs or other evidence of an intracranial lesion, these discount the diagnosis of cervical spondylosis. The hereditary ataxias do not show the remissions which are typical of disseminated sclerosis and they are often associated with bony deformity such as pes cavus and kyphoscoliosis.

Either delayed VERs or oligoclonal bands in the CSF are found in most cases of DS, but there is a group of patients in whom the diagnosis is suspected but will not be confirmed until the course of the illness is followed for several years.

Treatment

The cause of the disease is not known and there is at present no specific therapy. During an acute relapse the patient should rest in bed, although prolonged confinement to bed should be avoided as this encourages the development of spasticity. During remission he should be as active as possible while keeping within his own limits of exercise tolerance to avoid exhaustion. Mild intercurrent illness should be treated vigorously and the patient should protect himself from inclement weather.

The administration of corticosteroids seems to shorten a period of relapse. ACTH gel by injection is more effective, but in the high dosage necessary it can only be used in hospital under close medical supervision, and careful maintenance of electrolyte balance.

The care of the seriously disabled patient can be eased by the provision of appropriate mechanical aids, and is outlined in the section on paraplegia (p. 179).

TRANSVERSE MYELITIS

This is a complete or partial transverse inflammatory lesion of the spinal cord. The cause often remains unknown although it may be the first symptom of disseminated sclerosis or an incomplete form of acute disseminated encephalomyelitis.

Characteristically, the symptoms develop over a period of a few hours. In the initial stages of the disease there is a loss of sensation and a flaccid paralysis below the level of the lesion. This is accompanied by urinary retention and extensor plantar responses. There is usually some evidence of a sensory 'level' on the trunk and tenderness or hyperaesthesia at the upper limit of the sensory disorder.

There is also a progressive form of myelitis in which clinical deterioration continues during a period of 3 or 4 weeks. During this time the inflammatory process may spread longitudinally in the cord, causing respiratory embarrassment if the upper thoracic segments are affected, and complete respiratory paralysis if it reaches the third cervical segment.

Once the process becomes stationary there is a variable period before any improvement occurs. Some degree of recovery is usual. This may be complete, but more often there are some residua.

This condition should not be diagnosed unless spinal cord compression has been excluded by myelography.

NEUROMYELITIS OPTICA (Devic's disease)

Transverse myelitis occurring in conjunction with bilateral optic (retrobulbar) neuritis.

The eyes are often unequally affected so that there may be complete blindness in one eye while in the other, the vision seems hazy due to the presence of a central scotoma. The eye signs and myelitis may coincide or be separated by several weeks.

The prognosis for an individual attack is good, although there are usually some persistent stigmata and recurrent attacks may occur.

ACUTE DISSEMINATED ENCEPHALOMYELITIS

This is an uncommon consequence upon the viral exanthemata of childhood, vaccination against smallpox, and inoculation against rabies. A similar group of symptoms may present as the first episode in disseminated sclerosis.

The pathological findings which consist of numerous circumscribed areas of perivascular demyelination approximate to those which develop in experimental allergic encephalomyelitis in animals.

About one week after measles and ten days to two weeks after vaccination, there is a rapid development of neurological symptoms consisting of headache, drowsiness, stupor, ocular palsies and often a transverse cord lesion. The mortality rate is from 25–40 per cent, and patients who recover are frequently left with some disability, such as paraplegia or epilepsy.

Chapter 29
The Hereditary Ataxias

(Spinocerebellar degeneration)

This fairly uncommon group of disorders is typified by a familial incidence of ataxia developing in the second or third decade of life. The ataxia is commonly associated with other neurological signs such as spasticity, neuropathy, and optic atrophy. Skeletal malformations such as pes cavus and scoliosis are common. The progress of the disorder is usually gradual and the remissions typical of disseminated sclerosis are not experienced. There is considerable overlap between the different members of this group.

Friedreich's ataxia is the most commonly occurring example. The cerebellar signs, ataxia, nystagmus, intention tremor and slurred speech are combined with spastic paraplegia and diminished muscle/joint sensation. The plantar responses are extensor. The ankle jerks are lost early in the disease and as time passes the other tendon reflexes disappear. Pes cavus and cardiac fibromyopathy accompany the neurological signs. The constituents of the cerebrospinal fluid are normal.

Chapter 30
The Care of the Paraplegic Patient

The need for active and enthusiastic treatment is urgent. Prevention of the complications is less difficult than their cure. Immediate attention must be given to the care of the skin, the bladder, the patient's general condition and manipulation of the paralysed limbs.

The *skin* overlying bony protuberances is at particular risk in patients who are immobile and whose cutaneous sensation is impaired. Pressure sores can be prevented if the patient is turned at 2-hourly intervals night and day, and if the skin is kept clean, dry and powdered. Pressure on the ischial tuberosities, the trochanters, the sacrum and the heels is avoided by the use of sectioned sorbo-mattresses. Should a sore develop, the patient must be prevented from bearing any weight on it. A Stryker turning frame can be used to nurse him prone. Necrotic tissue should be trimmed away and slough encouraged to separate with eusol packs. Once clean, the sores should be exposed to the air and kept dry.

Bladder. After the acute onset of paraplegia the patient usually develops a retention of urine. At first the bladder is atonic. Emptying can sometimes be achieved by manual compression. More often, catheterization is required. This must be performed under conditions of strict asepsis. Infection should be treated by bladder lavage using a urinary antiseptic, and systemic antibiotics in full dosage for at least 10 days. Once the paraplegia is established it is possible to train an automatic bladder (p. 28) which can be emptied at regular intervals in response to abdominal pressure or some other voluntarily initiated reflex. Intramuscular or oral carbachol is of value in establishing control.

A twice-weekly enema is usually sufficient to maintain satisfactory bowel function.

The patient's *general condition* should be boosted with a high protein diet and if anaemia develops, transfusion with whole blood is of benefit.

The *limbs.* In the acute phase of the illness the legs should be moved passively to prevent the development of contractures. Heavy blankets should be lifted off the feet with a bed cage and splints provided to avoid foot drop deformities. When tone returns to the limbs, a skilled physiotherapist can utilize any surviving postural reflexes to enhance the extensor thrust of the legs so that weight can be borne. Every effort is made to give the paraplegic independence either by teaching him to walk with calipers and various types of support or by adapting him to an active wheelchair life.

There is no drug currently available which is fully effective in the relief of painful and incapacitating flexor spasms. Diazepam and baclofen give some measure of relief. Carefully controlled intrathecal injections of phenol can bring about a selective reduction in tone without affecting any remaining muscle power.

Chapter 31
Prolapsed Intervertebral Disc

The spinal column consists of a series of drum-like vertebral bodies separated by gelatinous intervertebral discs giving the column resilience and flexibility. The rib cage prevents any considerable movements of the thoracic spine and so the greater part of trunk flexion and rotation occurs in the lumbar region. The lumbar vertebrae also carry the total weight of the trunk, the head, the arms and any object which the patient may lift. With the spine erect, the structure of the vertebral bodies is ideally suited to this type of load. If the spine is flexed a severe strain is put on the posterior vertebral ligaments and there is a danger of posterior extrusion of the disc.

The herniation of a lumbar disc is usually preceded by a period of subacute backache, sometimes called lumbago. This is thought to be the result of minor injuries to the posterior vertebral ligaments, which are caused by faulty posture, awkward twisting movements of the spine or injudicious weight lifting. The final rupture of the vertebral ligament and the protrusion of the disc is often a dramatic event. The patient has bent down to do some unaccustomed lifting, when he feels something snap to his back, pain shoots down his leg and he is unable to straighten up. Later he finds that the pain is worsened by stooping or coughing or standing in any one position for a long period. He walks with great circumspection, holding his back rigidly.

The discs between the 4th and 5th lumbar vertebrae and the 5th lumbar and 1st sacral vertebrae are most often affected. The *lumbar 4–5 intervertebral disc* compresses the 5th lumbar nerve root. Pain is felt down the postero-lateral aspect of the thigh and leg and over the medial half of the foot. As only a single nerve root is involved, the sensory overlap from the adjacent roots usually minimizes any sensory loss, although there may be blunting of sensation over the lateral surface of the leg and dorsum of the foot. There is usually some weakness of dorsiflexion of the toes. The tendon reflexes are normal.

The *L5–S1 disc* compresses the 1st sacral root. Pain is felt more posteriorly down the thigh and leg and along the lateral border of the foot, where there may be blunting of sensation. Plantar flexion and eversion of the foot are weak and the ankle jerk is diminished.

The uncommon *L3–4 disc* prolapse involves the 4th lumbar nerve root, causing pain and numbness which extend down the lateral aspect of the thigh and crosses at the knee to the medial aspect of the leg. There is weakness of knee extension (quadriceps) and the knee jerk is diminished.

Examination of the back reveals a loss of the normal lumbar lordosis, with a variable scoliosis. The tilt may be away from the affected side, in a conscious effort to relieve the strain on the prolapsed disc, or towards the affected side due to muscle spasm. If the patient tries to touch his toes the rigidity of his back is more apparent, the scoliosis is exaggerated and the manoeuvre causes a worsening of the pain. Pressure over the affected disc space, a little lateral to the mid-line, also provokes pain.

Compression of the L5 or S1 nerve roots, results in a diminished straight leg raising test on the affected side. Flexion of the hip with the knee extended increases the tension on the displaced nerve root, causing pain in the back and reflex spasm of the ham-string muscles. In the case of a suspected L4 root lesion, the femoral stretch test may be of greater value. With the patient lying prone or on his side and with his leg held straight, the examiner attempts to hyperextend the hip. Pain and muscle spasm accompany a prolapsed L3–4 disc.

Investigation
Lateral and anteroposterior X-rays of the lumbar spine may show narrowing of the disc space and scoliosis. The CSF is often normal, but the protein content may be increased (0.5–0.8 g l^{-1}). The diagnosis can usually be made without recourse to myelography, but if surgical treatment is contemplated, a myelogram or radiculogram is normally obtained to confirm the localization.

Treatment
Strict bed rest on a hard mattress and without a pillow is the treatment during the acute phase of the illness. Analgesics should be given as required. Improvement in the straight leg raising test is the best indication of recovery. As the patient becomes free from pain he should undertake a course of back exercises to strengthen the sacrospinalis muscle.

During the period of supine bed rest, it is not uncommon for the patient to complain of dizziness. This resolves when he is remobilized.

Pain usually subsides within 3 or 4 weeks. The exercises should become part of the patient's daily routine. He should be instructed in the correct method of lifting, keeping his back upright.

Recurrent or persistent sciatica in the elderly is often relieved by wearing a spinal brace. Such symptoms in a younger patient are an indication for surgical treatment.

Prolapses of thoracic and cervical discs are relatively uncommon. **Thoracic disc** prolapse occurs at the site of pre-existing disease. If the affected disc is at D8–D10, straight X-rays usually show calcification there, while D11 and D12 discs are not usually calcified. A lateral prolapse causes girdle pain: a central prolapse causes cord compression. Surgical treatment, athough sometimes necessary is hazardous because of the precarious blood supply to the cord. Acute **cervical discs** are usually laterally placed, causing pain and a crick in the neck. They respond well to neck traction.

Cauda Equina Syndrome

A centrally placed lumbosacral disc or spondylolisthesis at the lumbosacral junction will compress the cauda equina, causing pain, sensory loss in the sacral region, weakness in the legs and loss of bladder control. Clinically, disc disease may be indistinguishable from tumours of the cauda equina such as ependymoma or neurofibroma.

Myelography and surgical treatment are urgently required to prevent irreversible damage.

Chapter 32
The Neuropathies

Diverse pathological conditions cause disorders of peripheral nerve function. The disorders which are associated with neuropathy may

be grouped conveniently according to their well-recognized properties.
1. Deficiency diseases.
2. Metabolic disorders.
3. Poisons.
4. Allergic manifestations.
5. Infections.
6. Inherited disorders.
7. Ischaemia.
8. Compression.

This does not imply a common pathological mechanism nor even a common anatomical site for the lesion.

A functional failure at the periphery of the nervous system may be due to disease of the parent cell within the spinal cord, or to disease along the peripheral course of the nerve. The nucleus of the cell is the most important site for neuronal metabolism and it is here that many pathological processes have their effect. The metabolic products are normally distributed along the peripheral axon and so a central metabolic disorder is manifest by peripheral dysfunction. Peripheral nerve conduction and nutrition also depend upon an intact myelin sheath and blood supply. Some neuropathies are truly peripheral in that they result from local primary demyelination or ischaemia.

Affections of the peripheral nerves may be divided into three broad symptom groups: polyneuropathy, radiculopathy and mononeuropathy.

Polyneuropathy

In this group the primary lesion is probably in the neurons and it would be more correct to call it a neuronopathy. The symptoms are first apparent at the ends of the longest nerves. There is axonal degeneration with 'die back'; recovery is by axonal regeneration. It is a slow process and often incomplete.

There is a symmetrical involvement of the two sides. Sometimes the legs are affected earlier and more severely than the arms. Sensory disturbances including paraesthesiae, dysaesthesiae and numbness first affect the tips of the fingers and toes, and then spread proximally, disregarding both segmental and peripheral nerve distribution. This is called glove and stocking sensory loss. The paraesthesiae are sometimes peculiarly unpleasant having a raw, burning quality. Pain and tenderness in the muscles and along the nerve trunks is not uncommon.

Weakness affects the distal muscles first, and later spreads proximally. Wasting occurs and the tone is decreased. The tendon reflexes are lost early in the disease, often before any weakness is apparent. The autonomic nerves are also affected causing trophic changes in the skin, loss of sweating and disordered vascular reflexes leading to postural hypotension. The constituents of the cerebrospinal fluid are usually normal.

The motor and sensory nerve fibres are often unequally involved in the pathological process. Not infrequently one function may remain apparently normal while the other is severely affected.

The deficiency diseases, metabolic disorders, and the poisons, give rise to this type of neuropathy.

Radiculopathy

The primary lesion is in the nerve roots proximal to their emergence through the intervertebral foramina. There is an initial demyelination with secondary axonal degeneration. The demyelination is thought to be the result of an allergic reaction. A similar condition may be induced in experimental animals by immunizing them with a boosted suspension of nerve tissue. As the disease presents in man, the role of an immunizing factor can be attributed to serum injections in the case of serum neuritis, or to preceding diphtheria causing delayed diphtheritic neuritis. On the other hand, the origin may be obscure as it is in the Guillain-Barré syndrome. The site of the lesion is within the subarachnoid space and there is a characteristic response in the cerebrospinal fluid. The protein is usually increased (up to 20 g l^{-1}) while there is little or no alteration in the number of cells (*Dissociation albuminocytologique*).

Sensory disorders are variable. In some instances, there is a segmental loss, but more often it is in the typical glove and stocking distribution. The sensation may be unaffected.

Weakness usually affects the proximal and distal limb muscles equally. Wasting occurs but is less prominent than in the polyneuropathies. The reflexes are usually diminished or absent.

Mononeuropathy

This is a local peripheral lesion resulting from infection, compression or ischaemic changes in a single nerve. There are both motor and sensory defects which are limited to the distribution of the affected nerve. Numerous, apparently separate, peripheral nerve lesions, resulting in an asymmetrical neuropathy, is called mononeuritis multiplex. This is a characteristic complication of the collagen vascular diseases.

DEFICIENCY DISEASES

Thiamine   Pyridoxine
Nicotinic acid   Cyanocobalamin
Pantothenic acid (Alcohol)

Deficiencies of thiamine, nicotinic acid and pantothenic acid interfere with neuronal metabolism by blocking the oxidation of glucose. Such a deficiency may result from malnutrition, vomiting, the increased demands of pregnancy, or the dietary perversions of the alcoholic. Thiamine deficiency may also give rise to cardiomyopathy and a haemorrhagic mid-brain encephalopathy (*Wernicke's encephalopathy*). This causes paralysis of ocular movements, nystagmus, ataxia and dementia. About a quarter of these patients develop the distinctive Korsakow syndrome, in which he confabulates to fill the gaps in his defective memory. The so-called alcoholic neuritis is due to a vitamin deficiency rather than the toxic effects of the alcohol. It is associated with a particularly severe calf pain.

Pellagra is due to a deficiency of nicotinic acid. In addition to the polyneuropathy, the patient may be mildly demented and show a distinctive dark, scaly dermatitis on the exposed areas of the body. There is commonly an accompanying glossitis and diarrhoea.

Pyridoxine (vitamin B6) deficiency results from prolonged treatment with isoniazid (INAH). It may also cause epileptic fits.

Cyanocobalamin (vitamin B12) deficiency is more completely described on p. 162. The majority of patients with megaloblastic anaemia have mild symptoms of peripheral neuropathy. The neuropathy may precede the development of anaemia.

METABOLIC DISORDERS

Diabetes mellitus   Amyloidosis
Porphyria   Carcinomatous neuropathy

Diabetes: neuropathy commonly accompanies long-standing, poorly controlled diabetes in the middle aged and elderly.

The most frequently occurring symptoms suggest a lesion in or near the posterior root ganglion. There is peripheral hypaesthesia with a profound loss of vibration sense. Pain is not universal but it may be disabling. Painless arthropathies, and trophic ulceration of the feet occur. The protein content of the cerebrospinal fluid is usually increased.

Diabetic amyotrophy is less common. It is a lower neuron weakness affecting the proximal limb muscles.

Autonomic involvement causes diarrhoea, postural hypotension, sweating and impotence.

Diabetic ischaemic mononeuropathy is due to atheromatous occlusion of the vasa nervorum. This is typically painful and most often affects the branches of the sciatic nerve, the median nerve and the third and sixth cranial nerves.

Porphyria: a relapsing asymmetrical motor neuropathy may accompany both acute and intermittent porphyria and porphyria cutanea tarda. Acute porphyria is often precipitated by barbiturates or alcohol and is accompanied by abdominal pain and mental disturbance.

They may be recognized during an acute phase by the excretion of porphobilinogen in the urine.

Carcinomatous neuropathy: the relationship between carcinoma and the neuropathy is not known. Both sensory and sensorimotor neuropathies occur. The protein content of the cerebrospinal fluid is often increased.

POISONS

The heavy metals, e.g. arsenic, gold, mercury and lead.

Organic substances, e.g. the industrial organic poisons, fat solvents, drugs, insecticides.

These are uncommon causes of neuropathy, but in the search for an aetiological agent, a careful inquiry should be made into the use of any drugs, solvents, chemicals or insecticides. With the exception of lead, the heavy metals inhibit the action of enzymes in the oxidation of glucose and so give rise to a neuropathy which is indistiguishable from that due to deficiency of the B group of vitamins.

Lead poisoning causes a motor neuropathy, especially affecting the radial, median and lateral popliteal nerves. Wrist drop and foot drop are the symptoms which occur most commonly. In this country lead paint is little used, but children may suffer from chewing imported lead painted toys or furniture.

Penicillamine and BAL are used in the treatment of heavy metal poisoning. These two drugs bind the metal in a non-toxic form until it is excreted in the urine.

Fat solvents. These may be absorbed through the skin or the fumes may be inhaled. Poisoning is usually a result of their use in industry. Their solvent properties may have a direct effect on the myelin of the peripheral nerves.

Insecticides. Some insecticides consist of long-acting anti-cholinesterases, which cause paralysis by cholinergic block. The onset of weakness is sudden and can be related to contact with the insecticide. The patient should be given atropine 1 mg IM and transferred to a centre where there are facilities for assisted respiration. The specific antidotes PAM or P2S are seldom available and of doubtful efficacy.

ALLERGIC MANIFESTATIONS

Guillain-Barré syndrome Serum neuritis
Late effects of diphtheritic infection Neuralgic amyotrophy

Guillain-Barré syndrome: The neurological symptoms are sometimes preceded by a mild flu-like illness and this disease used to be known as acute infective polyneuritis. Now this name has generally been discarded and it is considered to be due to a disordered immune response.

The motor symptoms are usually more prominent than the sensory loss. There is often a blunting of peripheral sensation in a glove and stocking distribution but sometimes the loss appears to be segmental. Both proximal and distal muscles are involved and the tendon reflexes are diminished. Pain in the shoulders and back is common. The facial and ocular muscles are frequently affected. An extension of the weakness of the muscles of the trunk to the thorax threatens respiration. While the disease is advancing, one should make frequent assessments of the patient's respiratory function. A satisfactory rough estimate can be made by asking the patient to take as big a breath as possible and then count. Most people reach 35 or 40 on one breath. At the first suggestion of respiratory failure or weakness of the 'bulbar' muscles, a tracheostomy should be performed, and with a cuffed tracheostomy tube intermittent positive pressure respiration instituted.

Untreated, the patient's condition usually deteriorates during the first few weeks of the illness. In the rapidly advancing cases (sometimes called Landry's paralysis) death results from respiratory failure. After a variable static period, there is a gradual improvement. Relapses and arrests are common. Most patients have some residual disability.

The cerebrospinal fluid contains an excess of protein (up to 20 g l^{-1}) but very few cells.

The deterioration can be checked and in some cases reversed if steroids are given within the first two or three weeks of the illness. Oral prednisolone, 60 mg daily, is effective in the mild cases, but ACTH gel 120 units daily should be given in any severe case. During the period of flaccid paralysis, the limbs should be supported so that overstretching of the muscles and tendons is prevented.

On occasions there may be cerebellar and upper motor neuron signs. This stresses the continuity of the spectrum of 'allergic' disorders from those involving the nerve roots (Guillain-Barré syndrome) to those involving the central nervous system (acute disseminated encephalomyelitis).

The delayed diphtheritic neuritis: six to eight weeks after diphtheria a symmetrical, primarily motor neuropathy may develop. This is in all ways similar to the Guillain-Barré syndrome and the cerebrospinal fluid shows the typical *dissociation albumino-cytologique*.

Neuralgic amyotrophy: severe pain in the shoulder and arm, followed by segmental weakness and sensory loss. It is usually unilateral, or if bilateral the involvement is asymmetrical. This condition may be identified with a preceding mild viral infection or it may develop *de novo*. One or two adjacent nerve roots are affected and there is occasionally an increase in the cellular and protein content of the cerebrospinal fluid. The numbness and pain usually resolve although the weakness may persist.

INFECTIONS

Leprosy and early diphtheritic neuritis

Leprosy is one of the few infections which affect the nerve directly. There is local thickening of the nerve at the site of infection, and the skin of the area supplied is depigmented and anaesthetic.

Diphtheria: the motor neuritis which sometimes occurs within 2 or 3 weeks of the initial infection is probably due to the local effect of toxins released by the organism. The palate, muscles of the pharynx, the facial muscles, and the intrinsic ocular muscles may be involved.

INHERITED DISORDERS

Peroneal muscular atrophy
Hypertrophic interstitial neuropathy

Great variations are to be found in these inherited neuropathies. In addition to the neuropathic signs there are bony stigmata such as pes cavus and spina bifida occulta, cerebellar signs and, occasionally, upper motor neuron signs.

Peroneal muscular atrophy: in spite of its name it is primarily a motor neuropathy affecting the distal muscles of the limbs. It is usually symmetrical and both legs and arms are affected. The proximal extension of the wasting seldom advances beyond the mid-thigh, so that the thighs have the characteristic appearance of inverted champagne bottles. There is almost always a loss of vibration sense at the ankles.

Hypertrophic interstitial neuropathy: This is a chronic motor polyneuropathy which rarely appears before middle age. The peripheral nerves are thickened. The ulnar nerve at the elbow and the lateral popliteal nerve at the knee are particularly easy to feel.

ISCHAEMIC NEUROPATHY

Thromboangiitis obliterans   Systemic lupus erythematosus
Polyarteritis nodosa   Diabetes mellitus
Rheumatoid arthritis

Mononeuritis multiplex is associated with several conditions which also cause an arteritis or arterial occlusion. Whether or not the relationship is causal is open to doubt. In the case of polyarteritis nodosa and systemic lupus erythematosus, allergic mechanisms and metabolic disorders may also be responsible.

COMPRESSION NEUROPATHIES

Carpal tunnel syndrome   Meralgia paraesthetica
Ulnar neuropathy

The compression of the spinal nerve roots has been discussed in the section on spondylosis (p. 158).

Carpal tunnel syndrome: the median nerve enters the palm of the hand in front of the tendons of the flexor digitorum sublimis and beneath the flexor retinaculum. This relatively confined space is called the carpal tunnel. The intrusion of fatty material or even oedema of the constituent parts causes a compressive median neuropathy. It may complicate pregnancy, obesity or myxoedema.

The symptoms consist of pain in the hands sometimes spreading proximally up the arm. The pain is worse at night, often waking the patient during the early hours of the morning. Paraesthesiae or numbness are experienced in the distribution of the median nerve and there is weakness and wasting of the muscles of the thenar eminence, excepting the adductor pollicis. The abductor pollicis brevis is affected early, giving rise to a characteristic wasting of the antero-lateral border of the thenar eminence. The symptoms are worsened by heavy manual work such as laundering or scrubbing.

Relief is obtained by splinting the wrist at night on a moulded polythene splint. If the precipitating condition is not likely to respond to treatment, then it is usually necessary to relieve pressure on the nerve by dividing the flexor retinaculum.

Ulnar neuropathy: the ulnar nerve is particularly exposed to injury at the elbow. Ulnar neuropathy may result from the late effects of fracture dislocations of the medial epicondyle of the humerus. Such a lesion causes weakness of wrist flexion, of the flexors of the ring and little fingers, of adduction and abduction of the fingers and adduction of the thumb. There is a loss of cutaneous sensation over the hypothenar eminence, the little finger and the ulnar half of the ring finger. The symptoms are relieved by a surgical transplant of the nerve to the anterior aspect of the elbow.

The ulnar nerve may be involved in a compressive lesion in the palm of the hand. Injury to the nerve may be due to a manual workers occupation or to weight bearing on a walking stick. The flexor carpi ulnaris and the flexor digitorum profundis which receive their innervation in the forearm are not affected. Cutaneous sensation similarly escapes. Otherwise the weakness will be like that described in the previous paragraph.

Meralgia paraesthetica: the lateral cutaneous nerve of the thigh leaves the pelvis beneath the inguinal ligament and then penetrates the fascia lata before surfacing on the lateral aspect of the thigh. Obesity and pregnancy may both cause entrapment of the nerve at these two sites. The symptoms are of painful paraesthesiae down the outer aspect of the thigh, with diminished cutaneous sensation. The symptoms are aggravated by walking and relieved by rest.

Treatment of Neuropathies

Treatment is aimed at the correction of any of the apparent abnormalities, e.g. restoration of normal nutrition; supplements of deficient vitamins; treatment of diabetes; relief of compression, etc.

For those conditions thought to be due to a disordered immune reaction, steroids are currently used.

General measures during the acute or advancing phase of the illness include: bed rest, support of the paralysed parts (using splints if necessary), analgesics for the relief of pain, maintenance of good nutrition.

As recovery begins the physiotherapist should supervise the patient's rehabilitation.

Chapter 33
Myasthenia Gravis

This illness is characterized by the abnormally rapid onset of weakness during sustained or repeated contraction of the muscles. Unlike normal fatiguability, the myasthenic weakness may be so extreme as to cause complete paralysis. The weakness recovers after a period of rest and responds to the administration of anti-cholinesterase drugs.

Aetiology. The arrival of a motor impulse at the prejunctional nerve ending discharges acetylcholine from the storage vesicles there. This diffuses across the neuromuscular junction and creates sufficient energy to initiate an action potential in the post-junctional motor end plate. In the myasthenic patient, the quanta of acetylcholine are abnormally small and are readily exhausted. The acetylcholine receptors are reduced in number and their function is impaired by immunological damage mediated by circulating antibodies. Cholinesterase breaks down the acetylcholine to release choline which itself may intensify the neuromuscular block by competitive inhibition. Continuing effort is accompanied by increasing weakness.

Abnormal aggregations of lymphocytes are commonly found in the thymus glands of patients suffering from myasthenia gravis. The lymphocytes appear to be formed in germinal centres scattered through the gland. The thymus may be enlarged but is usually of normal size, and actual thymic tumours are found in less than a fifth of cases. The presence of germinal centres suggests that the thymic activity is part of a generalized response of the reticulo-endothelial system to a foreign protein. Myasthenia gravis is sometimes associated with diseases which are commonly considered to be due to an auto-immune reaction, e.g. thyroid disorders and rheumatoid arthritis.

Easy fatiguability of specific muscles is the key to the diagnosis of myasthenia, and as might be expected, the symptoms are usually more prominent at the end of the day.

Not all the muscles are equally affected. The eye muscles are most frequently involved, causing a variable ptosis and diplopia. Sometimes the disease appears to remain limited to this area (ocular myasthenia), but more often it is accompanied by weakness elsewhere in the body. The muscles of mastication and deglutition are the next most commonly affected, after which come the muscles of the face, the neck, the shoulders, the pelvic girdle, limbs and trunk. Involvement of the respiratory muscles is a serious hazard, as under normal circumstances there is no prospect of resting them.

There are fluctuations in the severity of the disease and long periods of remission are common. Relapses are ascribed to inter-current infection, trauma, and psychological stress. The careful management of a patient during a relapse is often rewarded by remission. Women are most often affected during their reproductive life, but men may develop the disease at any age.

Physical examination should include the effects of fatigue, for at rest a mildly affected patient may appear normal. In addition to this, a test dose of an anticholinesterase drug is used in diagnosis. Preceded by 0·6 mg atropine subcutaneously, 0·5–1·0 mg of neostigmine is given subcutaneously. The patient is examined at 15-minute intervals up to 1 hour. The maximum effect is usually seen between 30 minutes and 1 hour. It is essential that objective measurements should be made before and during the test as the patient's subjective response is unreliable. Edrophonium chloride 10 mg IV is also used as a diagnostic agent, but its action is so brief that the effect may be missed.

Treatment
Neostigmine and pyridostigmine are the drugs of choice. The ideal dose for any patient is a matter for careful experiment. When several muscle groups are involved it is likely that the dosage which

is ideal for some muscles will cause overdosage effects in others. Overdosage causes weakness due to persistent depolarization of the muscle membrane. When a patient becomes increasingly weak and no longer responds to his drugs, one should suspect an overdosage effect. The signs of overdosage are:

(a) in the muscles: weakness and fasciculation;

(b) on the parasympathetic system: hypersalivation, abdominal cramps; borborygmi and diarrhoea, sweating and meiosis.

If the patient is overdosed, all anticholinesterase medication must be withdrawn. If respiration is embarrassed, a tracheostomy and assisted respiratory may be necessary.

Parasympathetic side effects are sometimes present even when the patient is ideally dosed. In this case atropine may be given routinely to counteract them, remembering that signs of true overdosage may be obscured.

Thymectomy. In selected patients, thymectomy seems to bring about an earlier and more complete remission than might otherwise be expected. Young women, with increasing disability and within the first five years of the onset of the disease, get the most benefit.

Steroids, although often causing a temporary worsening of the myasthenia, may induce a remission when a course of treatment is complete. This treatment should only be given with the patient in hospital so that any deterioration may be recognized and treated.

The myasthenic patient is especially sensitive to curare and other neuromuscular blocking agents including the antibiotics streptomycin and gentamycin.

Plasmapheresis provides a method of removing antibodies and immune complexes from the circulation. This is usually accompanied by clinical improvement. It must be combined with immunosuppressives to prevent a rebound increase in the circulating antibodies.

The myasthenic (Eaton-Lambert) syndrome is most often found in association with bronchial carcinoma. There is a failure of acetylcholine release at the neuromuscular junction. The syndrome may be distinguished from true myasthenia gravis by electromyography. Tetanization of the nerve facilitates the release of acetylcholine and the amplitude of the motor units increases. Guanidine 20 mg/kg/day may relieve the symptoms.

Chapter 34
Diseases of the Muscle

Wasting and weakness of the muscles may be due to disease of the lower motor neuron, when it is called neurogenic atrophy, or it may be due to a primary disease of the muscles. This is known as a myopathy. Myopathy may be inherited or acquired. Inherited myopathy is called muscular dystrophy. Acquired myopathies include the inflammatory diseases of muscle (myositis or polymyositis), muscle disease associated with thyrotoxicosis, steroid administration and the collagen–vascular disorders, and muscle disease which occurs as a non-metastatic complication of visceral carcinoma.

The differentiation of the myopathies depends on:
1. A complete clinical description of the disorder, with details of the age at onset, the distribution of weakness and its rate of progression.
2. A family history of muscle disease.
3. Electromyography for distinguishing between neurogenic atrophy and primary disease of the muscle.
4. Biochemical estimation of the muscle enzymes in the circulating blood. The finding of greatly increased amounts of creatine kinase in the blood is a feature of Duchenne dystrophy and myositis.
5. Muscle biopsy. This is of value in differentiating muscular dystrophy and myositis.

Muscular dystrophy: In a single section both normal and abnormal fibres are seen. The affected fibres first swell and their contents become cloudy. These fibres then degenerate and the atrophic fibres are replaced by fatty tissue. Fine spindly fibres are sometimes seen. There is practically no regeneration.

Myositis: The degeneration of muscle fibres is more diffuse. The cross striations disappear and there is active phagocytosis of degenerating muscle fibres. The fibres are separated by oedema, and there are striking lymphocytic infiltrations around the blood vessels.

MUSCULAR DYSTROPHY

Clinically, the muscle weakness and wasting occurs in a selective distribution. The tendon reflexes are diminished. There is no fasciculation. The muscles are not tender. There are no sensory abnormalities. As yet there is no proven method of treatment. The classification of this group of inherited disorders is primarily descriptive.
1. Duchenne dystrophy.
2. Facio-scapulo-humeral dystrophy.
3. Limb-girdle dystrophy.
4. Muscular dystrophy accompanied by myotonia.
5. Rarer types of muscular dystrophy.

Duchenne dystrophy

This is almost entirely restricted to boys. It begins early in life, usually before the age of four, but occasional cases have appeared in the second and third decade (Becker X-linked dystrophy).

The earliest signs are of symmetrical weakness and wasting of the muscles of the pelvic girdle and the back. This makes the child walk with a waddling gait and an exaggerated lumbar lordosis. It also makes him rise to his feet in a characteristic way. From lying on his back, he first rolls over on to his face. He takes up a crouching posture, and then straightens his legs. He pushes himself upright by 'climbing hand over hand up his legs'. This manoeuvre is not in itself diagnostic of Duchenne dystrophy. Pseudohypertrophy of the calves is commonly seen. The calf muscles are not involved in the dystrophic process until late in the disease.

The degenerative process is steadily and often rapidly progressive. It extends to the shoulders and upper limbs within a few years. Not all muscles are equally affected and the distribution of wasting allows the still-active muscles to shorten and develop contractures. Within ten years the patient can seldom walk and long periods of immobility cause osteoporosis and skeletal deformity. Death due to respiratory infection or cardiac failure usually occurs before the age of twenty.

In the early and acute stages of the disease the serum creatine kinase is greatly increased. Duchenne dystrophy is inherited as a sex-linked recessive character. In a large proportion of cases the mother of an affected child also has a raised serum creatine kinase. The enzyme may be evident in the blood of clinically unaffected siblings. The disease is uncommonly inherited in an autosomal recessive form, accounting for its rare appearance in girls.

Although there is no curative treatment the burden of the disability can be eased with physiotherapy, various orthopaedic measures to overcome contractions, and a suitable diet to prevent obesity.

Facio-scapulo-humeral dystrophy

The essential diagnostic feature is the early involvement of the muscles of the face. Males and females are equally affected, and although the disease may appear in childhood, it is more often delayed until the second or third decade. The onset is typically insidious and there may be indefinitely long periods of arrest. The involvement of the face, shoulders and arms is often asymmetrical and the spread to the muscles of the lower limb seldom occurs until 20 or 30 years after the onset. Pseudohypertrophy, deformity and gross disability are uncommon. Raised serum levels of the muscle enzymes are rarely found due to the slow progression of the disease.

It is inherited as an autosomal dominant factor.

Limb-girdle dystrophy

The disease affects males and females equally, the age at onset being from adolescence to middle life. If the early signs are found in the shoulder girdle then, like facio-scapulo-humeral dystrophy the weakness is often asymmetrical, the progression is slow and pseudohypertrophy is rare. If the pelvic girdle muscles are first affected then the progress of the disease is likely to be more acute, it is more often symmetrical and pseudohypertrophy is occasionally seen. In these respects it mimics Duchenne dystrophy. Like the uncommon sub-variety of Duchenne dystrophy it is inherited as an autosomal recessive. Difficulty may be experienced in distinguishing limb-girdle dystrophy from spinal muscular atrophy (p. 168).

Muscular dystrophy, accompanied by myotonia

Myotonia is a condition of heightened excitability of the muscle membrane. Muscular contraction is self-perpetuating with the result that the patient has difficulty in relaxing the muscle after an especially vigorous contraction. Myotonia may also be elicited by percussing the muscle with a tendon hammer or by direct mechanical stimulation of the muscle during electromyography.

Myotonia may be apparent in early childhood. This is called *myotonia congenita*. It is equally common in males and females and occurs in several generations of the same family. The affected child is stiff and slow in initiating movements. His muscles are often hypertrophied but weakness is not prominent. As he grows older the myotonia becomes less apparent, but on rare occasions the child with myotonia congenita has developed a dystrophy in later life.

Dystrophia myotonica. In this form, the muscle wasting is usually more prominent than the myotonia. Both males and females are affected and it appears in early middle age.

Characteristically, the facial muscles, the muscles of mastication and the sternomastoid muscles are affected early in the disease. This gives rise to a rather gaunt appearance, with drooping eyelids, slightly open mouth and a long, thin neck. In the limbs the distal muscles are more severely affected than the proximal ones. Voluntary myotonia may be demonstrated by asking the patient to grasp some small object in his hand. When told to 'let go' there is an appreciable delay before the finger flexors relax.

Percussion myotonia may be elicited in the extensor muscles of the forearm, the abductors of the thumb and the tongue. In response to a sharp tap on the belly of the muscle with a tendon hammer, there is a brisk contraction, then a delay before relaxation occurs.

Gonadal atrophy, frontal baldness and lenticular cataract, are common. Clinically unaffected siblings and parents may bear these stigmata. Personality disorders occur frequently.

X-rays of the skull show a small bridged pituitary fossa and a thick bony vault.

It is inherited as an autosomal dominant.

Treatment

Myotonia can be minimized by giving procaine amide 0·25 g four times a day up to a maximum of 4 g a day, diphenylhydantoin 100 mg three or four times a day, or quinine sulphate 0·3–0·6 g three times a day.

The rarer types of muscular dystrophy

Ocular myopathy: For many years the weakness remains limited to ocular muscles, but eventually the limb muscles are involved. Degenerative changes are sometimes found in the retina.

Distal myopathy: a very rare form of muscular dystrophy affecting the distal muscles of the limbs and later spreading proximally.

Congenital myopathy: a gradually progressive myopathy which is evident at birth.

ACQUIRED MYOPATHY

Polymyositis

Polymyositis is a symptom complex rather than a specific disease. The onset may be acute or subacute, and it sometimes persists for several years. The proximal limb muscles are symmetrically involved, without the selective sparing which occurs in muscular dystrophy. At the onset, the affected muscles are swollen and tender, and wasting is not prominent unless the disease enters a chronic phase. Occasionally it may be limited to a single muscle group, such as the muscles of the anterior compartment of the leg. There may be features which suggest that this is one of the collagen–vascular diseases such as Raynaud's phenomenon, joint disease, a high ESR, and abnormal gamma globulins in the blood. The skin overlying the affected muscles may be oedematous, reddened and atrophic. This presentation is called *dermatomyositis*.

Not all cases have florid evidence of inflammation and it is difficult to differentiate the chronic phase of this disease from limb-girdle dystrophy. Without treatment the acute form often advances to involve the respiratory muscles and causes death. Spontaneous remissions may occur in the acute and subacute varieties, although the latter more often enter a chronic phase.

Diagnosis. The muscle enzymes are usually elevated. EMG shows myopathic features although these are sometimes mixed with elements normally associated with neuropathy. A positive biopsy may result only after careful and possibly repeated examination.

Treatment

During the acute phase of this illness the patient should remain in bed. Steroids are used in the symptomatic treatment. ACTH seems to be more rapidly effective than oral steroids, but is not otherwise to be preferred. Prednisolone 60 mg daily is given initially for two weeks, after which the dose may be gradually reduced. Repeated estimations of the S. creatine kinase are of value for predicting the course of the disease and for adjusting the steroid dosage. Withdrawal of steroids is attended by the risk of relapse. It is sometimes necessary to keep the patient on a maintenance dose for several months. The lowest dose which will prevent relapse should be used. Immunosuppressives and thymectomy are sometimes employed.

'Late-life' myopathy

Myopathy developing in late middle age seldom has any features of inflammatory disease. The muscles are not tender and the ESR is normal. There is a gradual deterioration with periods of arrest. In men a proportion of these cases is associated with malignant disease, whereas in women the cause often remains obscure. The age of the patients has suggested the term 'menopausal dystrophy'.

Metabolic myopathy

The use of systemic triamcinolone occasionally caused a non-tender proximal myopathy. It resolved when the offending drug was withdrawn and replaced with prednisolone. In the future it may appear with other steroids. In Cushing's syndrome a similar myopathy is sometimes seen.

Thyrotoxic myopathy

This proximal myopathy is sometimes quite severe when the thyrotoxicosis is mild or clinically inapparent. Fasciculation is often seen in the affected muscles. It responds to treatment of the underlying disorder.

Carcinomatous myopathy

The relationship between myopathy and visceral carcinoma is poorly understood. The rate of progression and severity of the two conditions seems to be unrelated. It should be considered in the differential diagnosis of any myopathy developing in middle age.

DISORDERS OF POTASSIUM UTILIZATION

Disorders of potassium utilization results in intermittent weakness without any gross structural abnormality of the muscle.

Familial periodic paralysis: During an attack there is profound weakness of the limb muscles, and the serum potassium falls to less than 3 mEq/l. This is due to the migration of potassium into the cells. It may be provoked by a large carbohydrate meal and the consequent release of insulin. Attacks are most common after a period of rest and occur typically in the early morning. Each attack is usually self-limiting, but will be shortened by the administration of oral potassium. It is a disorder of young men and women and usually remits before the age of thirty.

Spontaneously occurring hyperkalaemia causes a similar flaccid paralysis. This is called *adynamia episodica hereditaria*. An attack may be provoked by giving oral potassium and relieved by giving intravenous calcium. It appears in early childhood.

THE 'FLOPPY BABY'

Muscular weakness and hypotonia in children under one year old may be due to:
1. Cerebral palsy.
2. Infantile motor neuron disease.
3. Kugelberg Welander atrophy.
4. Congenital myopathy.
5. Benign congenital hypotonia.

A proportion of children who will eventually develop spastic or athetoid cerebral palsy may present in the early months of life with flaccid limbs. The more characteristic disorders of tone appear when the postural reflexes would normally be developed. EMG, muscle biopsy, and muscle enzymes are normal.

Infantile motor neuron disease (Werdnig-Hoffman disease) appears soon after birth. It is a progressive condition characterized by muscular wasting, weakness, hypotonia and fasciculation. The EMG is diagnostic. Death occurs in 3–4 years. The Kugelberg Welander atrophy is a very slowly progressive condition first appearing in childhood and compatible with a normal life expectancy. There is wasting and weakness of the proximal limb muscles: it is primarily a neuronal disorder.

Congenital myopathy presents with wasting and weakness of the proximal limb muscles at birth. It is a familial disorder. Gradual deterioration occurs leading to death after 4 or 5 years.

A completely benign form of congenital hypotonia is sometimes seen. Moderate generalized weakness and hypotonicity is present at birth in the baby then gradually improves, eventually to become completely normal.

Chapter 35
The Non-Metastatic Complications of Carcinoma

Carcinoma of the lung, and less often carcinoma of the stomach, bowel, uterus and ovary are associated with neurological complications. They are not due to macroscopic metastases and it has been variously suggested that they are the result of a conditioned metabolic deficiency, infection, a secondary toxicity or a tissue sensitization.

The most frequently occurring neurological complication is a symmetrical sensory neuropathy. Subacute cerebellar degeneration, mixed motor and sensory neuropathy, myopathy and cerebral atrophy with dementia, also occur. The neurological signs usually precede the symptoms due to the tumour, and their rate of development seems to bear little relationship to its malignancy.

In the cerebellar degeneration, the cerebrospinal fluid often contains an excess of protein, and a first-zone gold curve.

The myopathy sometimes mimics myasthenia gravis. There is an abnormal 'fatiguability' of the affected muscles, and a partial response to anticholinesterase drugs. In this condition, unlike true myasthenia gravis, the eye muscles and the bulbar muscles are seldom affected and there is often a profound areflexia. The early response to anticholinesterase drugs is soon lost.

Suggestions for Further Reading

FEILLING A. ed. (1951) *Modern Trends in Neurology*, Vol. I. Butterworth, London.

HAYMAKER W. (1969) *Bing's Local Diagnosis in Neurological Diseases*, translated from the 15th German edition. Henry Kimpton, London.

JENNETT W.B. (1977) *An Introduction to Neurosurgery*, 3rd ed. Heinemann, London.

MERRITT H. HOUSTON. (1979) *A Textbook of Neurology*, 6th ed. Henry Kimpton, London.

NORMAN R.M. *et. al.* (1963) *Greenfields Neuropathology*, 2nd ed. Edward Arnold, London.

WALTON J.N. ed. (1969) *Disorders of Voluntary Muscle*, 2nd ed. J. & A. Churchill, London.

WILLIAMS D. ed. (various dates) *Modern Trends in Neurology*, Vols. II, III, IV, V and VI.

Index

Abdominal reflexes 78
Abducens nerve 33, 68
Abscess, brain 108 *et seq.*
Accessory motor cortex 45, 91
Accommodation (convergence) reflex 35
Acetylcholine 6, 7, 24, 193
Achlorhydria, gastric 163
Acoustic nerve tumour 104
Acromegaly 105
Actomycin 8
Adenoma, chromophobe 105
Adenosine triphosphate (ATP) 8
Adversive attacks 91
Adynamia episodica hereditaria 202
Agnosia, auditory 61
   tactile (astereognosis) 46
Agraphia 46
Akathisia 139
Alcoholic neuritis 186
Allergic reactions in the nervous system 172, 178, 184, 188
Alzheimer's disease 135
Amaurosis fugax 124
Amnesia 62, 98
Amyotrophic lateral sclerosis 166
Amyotrophy, diabetic 187
   neuralgic 190
   syphilitic 114
Anaemia, megaloblastic 163
Aneurysm 51, 127
Angiography 107, 130
Angioma 129
Anhydrosis 25
Anosmia 29, 104
Anterior cerebral artery 51, 124
Anticholinergic drugs 138
Anticonvulsants 93
Aphasia 61
Apraxia 11, 46
Argyll Robertson pupil 35, 116
Arnold-Chiari malformation 169
Arteries, intracranial, distribution 50
   occlusion 124
   stenosis 122
   spinal 53, 160

Arteriosclerosis, cerebral 123
Arteriovenous anomaly 129
Arteritis, syphilitic 113
   temporal 146
Arthropathy 115
Aseptic sinus thrombosis 131
Associated movements 14, 137
Astereognosis 46
Astrocytoma 103
Ataxia, cerebellar 79
   Friedreich's 179
   frontal 45
   hereditary 155, 179
   sensory 79
Athetosis 14, 96, 140
Atrophy, muscular 9, 196
   peroneal 190
   progressive 167
   optic 33, 116, 132, 164, 174, 179
Audiometry 71
Auditory meatus, internal 40, 105
Auditory nerve 40, 70
Aura, epileptic 88
   migrainous 144
Autonomic nervous system 23

Basal ganglia 12 *et seq.*, 47, 136 *et seq.*
Basilar artery 52, 124, 145
Bell's palsy 149
Biopsy, muscle 196
Birth injury 95, 161
Bladder 26, 100, 174, 180
Blood-brain barrier 56
Body image 46, 76
Bradykinesia 13, 137
Brain death 101
Brain injury 97 *et seq.*
Brain-stem 47
Broca's area 61
Brown-Séquard syndrome 55, 157
Bruit 124, 129
Bulbar palsy 167

Caloric tests 72
Capsule, internal 9, 12

Index

Carcinoma, non-metastatic complications 187, 203
Carcinomatous myopathy 202
Carcinomatous neuropathy 187
Carotid artery 51
  internal 50, 51, 124
Carpal tunnel syndrome 191
Cataplexy 85
Cauda equina 53
  syndrome 183
Causalgia 25
Cavernous sinus 131
Centrencephalic epilepsy 85, 88
Cephalgia, histaminic 148
Cerebellum 15, 77, 175
Cerebrospinal fluid 55, 175
Cerebrovascular disease 122 et seq.
Cervical rib 162
Cervical spondylosis 153, 158
Charcot joint 115, 170
Chiasm, optic 30
Cholinesterase 7, 193
Chorda tympani 40
Chorea 14, 140
  Huntington's 135, 141
  Sydenham's 141
Choriomeningitis, acute lymphocytic 121
Circle of Willis 50, 124, 127
Clasp knife phenomenon 18
Clonus 77
Cochlea 40, 42
Cochlear nerve 42
Colloidal gold curve 56
Compressive lesions 59
Computerized axial tomography 107
Concomitant strabismus 36
Concussion 58, 97
Conduction deafness 70
Confrontation 67
Coning 57
Conjugate eye movements 33
Consciousness 58
Conus medullaris 52
Convergence 35
Convulsions 92
Co-ordination 11, 76
Copper metabolism 139
Cord shock 54
Corneal reflex 69
Corpora quadrigemina 30
Cortex, cerebral 3, 11, 45
Corti, organ of 42

Cracked pot sound 101
Cranial nerves 48, 66 et seq.
Craniopharyngioma 106
Creatine 8, 196
Cremasteric reflex 78
Cyanocobalamin 134, 163, 186
Cystometry 27

Deafness 43, 70, 151
Deficiency diseases 186
Degeneration, spinocerebellar 179
  subacute combined 154, 162
Déja vu 92
Delirium 133
Dementia 116, 132 et seq., 164
Demyelinating diseases 172 et seq.
Denticulate ligaments 52
Dermatomyositis 200
Devic's disease 178
Diabetes mellitus 59, 187
Diphtheria 190
Diphtheritic neuritis 189
Diplopia 36, 68, 175
Disc, intervertebral 158, 181
Disc, optic 29, 67
Disseminated sclerosis 155, 172 et seq.
Dissociation albumino-cytologique 185
Doll's head manoeuvre 80
Drop attacks 84
Drug-induced movement disorder 138
Duchenne dystrophy 197
Dysaesthesiae 19
Dysarthria 60
Dysdiadochokinesia 16
Dyskinesias 139
Dysmetria 16
Dysphasia 60
Dyssynergia 175
Dystonia 14
Dystrophia myotonica 199
Dystrophy, muscular 196 et seq.

Eaton-Lambert syndrome 195
Edinger-Westphal nucleus 34
Electroencephalography 89, 92, 107
Embolism, cerebral 125
Encephalitis, acute 108
  virus 120
Encephalomyelitis, acute disseminated 178

Index

Encephalopathy, hypertensive 130
  Wernicke's 133, 186
Endarteritis obliterans 114
Enophthalmos 25
Ependymoma 103, 104
Epilepsia partialis continuans 90
Epilepsy 59, 83 *et seq*., 100, 135
Epilepsy, treatment 93
Erb's palsy 161
Euphoria 175
Extrapyramidal system 3, 4

Facial nerve 39, 69
Facial pain 146
Facial palsy 149
Facio-scapulo-humeral dystrophy 198
Familial periodic paralysis 202
Fasciculation 9, 166
Fasciculus, medial longitudinal 41, 48
Fat solvents 188
Fibrillation 10
Floppy baby 202
Focal epilepsy 90
Friedreich's ataxia 179
Froin's syndrome 157
Fundoscopy 67

Gait 79
Gamma globulin 57
General paresis (GPI) 116
Geniculate body, lateral 30
  medial 43
Geniculate ganglion 40
  herpes 150
Gerstmann's syndrome 46
Giant cell arteritis 146
Gigantism 105
Glabellar tap 38
Glioblastoma 103
Glossopharyngeal nerve 43, 70, 72
Glove and stocking 184
Grand mal 88
Grasp reflex 45
Guillain-Barré syndrome 188

Haematoma 98
Haemotomyelia 171
Haemorrhage, cerebral 125
  extradural 98
  subdural 98
  subarachnoid 127
Hallucination 84

Head injury 58, 134
Headache 142 *et seq.*
Hearing, tests of 70
Heavy metals and neuropathy 188
Hemianopia 30, 105, 128
Hemiballismus 14
Hemiplegia 96
Hemispasticity 79
Hepato-lenticular degeneration 139
Hereditary ataxia 155, 179
Herpes simplex 120
Herpes zoster 120, 150
Histaminic cephalgia 148
Holmes-Adie syndrome 36
Horner's syndrome 25
Huntington's chorea 135, 141
Hydrocephalus 56
Hydrocephalus, normal pressure 135
Hyperacusis 150
Hyperostosis 104
Hyperpituitarism 105
Hypertension, benign intracranial 132
Hypertensive encephalopathy 130
Hypertrophic interstitial neuropathy 191
Hypnagogic hallucinations 84
Hypoglossal nerve 44, 73
Hypoglycaemia 84, 134
Hypopituitarism 105
Hypothalamus 23, 47
Hypothyroidism 134
Hypotonia 18
Hypsarrhythmia 93
Hysterical fits 85

Infantile spasms 93
Infarction 123
Insecticides 188
Insulin 84
Intention tremor 16
Internal carotid artery 124
Intervertebral disc, prolapsed 181 *et seq.*
Intoxication 59
Intracranial hypertension, benign 132
Intracranial pressure, raised 57, 102
Involuntary movements 14
Ischaemic neuropathy 191
Isoniazid (INAH) 112, 186

Jacksonian seizure 90

Jamais vu 92
Jargon aphasia 61
Jaw jerk 38, 69

Kayser Fleischer ring 139
Kernicterus 96, 140
Kernig's test 75
Klumpke's paralysis 162
Korsakow syndrome 186
Kugelberg-Welander syndrome 168, 203

Labyrinth 41
Labyrinthine vertigo 151
Labyrinthitis 152
Laceration, cerebral 98
Landry's paralysis 189
Lange curve 56
Lateral sinus 131
Lead 188
Lemniscus, medial 48
Leprosy 190
Levodopa 138
Lhermitte's sign 174
Light reflex 34
Limb-girdle dystrophy 198
Limbs, examination 73
Lumbago 181
Lumbar puncture 53, 112, 128
Lymphocytic choriomeningitis 121

Macula 68
Medulloblastoma 104
Meiosis 25
Memory 61
Ménière's disease 151
Meningeal irritation 142
Meningioma 104, 157
Meningitis, acute purulent 110
  bacterial 110 et seq.
  meningococcal 110
  secondary 111
  tuberculous 112
Meningovascular syphilis 113, 154
Menopausal myopathy 201
Meralgia paraesthetica 192
Metabolic myopathy 201
Middle cerebral artery 52, 124
Middle ear deafness 43
Migraine 143 et seq.
Migrainous neuralgia 148
Miner's nystagmus 37
Mononeuritis multiplex 186, 191

Mononeuropathy 186
Motor aphasia 61
Motor cortex 3, 45, 90
Motor end plate 6
Motor neuron, lower 9
  upper 5, 8
Motor neuron disease 154, 165, 203
Muscle fibre 7, 8, 10
Muscle spindle 17
Muscle tone 16
Muscular atrophy—see atrophy
Muscular dystrophy 196 et seq.
Myasthenia gravis 10, 193 et seq., 204
Myasthenic syndrome 195
Myelitis, transverse 155, 177
Myoclonic epilepsy 90
Myoclonus 14
Myopathy 196 et seq.
  acquired 200
  carcinomatous 202
  congenital 200, 203
  distal 206
  late-life 201
  menopausal 201
  metabolic 201
  ocular 200
  thyrotoxic 201
Myositis 196
Myotonia 199

Narcolepsy 84
Nasopharyngeal carcinoma 147
Neck, examination 73, 160
Necrotizing encephalitis 120
Nerve deafness 43, 70
Neuralgia, migrainous 148
  post-herpetic 121, 148
  trigeminal 147
Neuralgic amyotrophy 190
Neurofibroma 157
Neuromuscular junction 6, 9, 193
Neuromyelitis optica 178
Neuron 3
Neuropathy 183 et seq.
Neurosyphilis 113 et seq.
Nicotinic acid 186
Nominal aphasia 61
Nucleus ambiguus 49
Nucleus pulposus 158
Nystagmus 16, 36, 72, 175

Occipital lobe 47

Index

Oculomotor nerve 33, 68
Oedema, cerebral 57, 98, 130
Olfactory groove meningioma 104
Olfactory nerve 29, 66
Ophthalmic artery 51
Ophthalmoplegic migraine 145
Ophthalmoscopy 67
Optic nerve 29 et seq., 66
Osteophytes 158

Paget's disease 148
Palaeocerebellum 15
Palsy, Bell's 149
  bulbar 167
  cerebral 95 et seq.
  Erb's 161
  facial 149
  pseudobulbar 9, 168
  progressive supranuclear 137
Pancoast's superior sulcus tumour 162
Papilloedema 32, 57, 67, 132
Paradoxical embolism 108
Paraesthesiae 19, 174, 184
Paralysis, familial periodic 202
  general, of the insane 116, 134
  Klumpke's 162
  Landry's 189
  Todd's 90
Paralytic strabismus 36
Paraplegia 54, 96, 179 et seq.
Parasympathetic system 25
Parenchymatous neurosyphilis 114
Parietal lobe 21, 46, 76
Parkinsonism 79, 136 et seq.
Pellagra 186
Perimetry 67
Peripheral nerve 6, 19, 183
Perlia, nucleus of 34
Peroneal muscular atrophy 190
Petit mal 89
Pick's disease 135
Pituitary tumour 105
Plantar reflex 18, 78
Plasmapheresis 195
Plexiform neuroma 158
Pneumoencephalography 107
Poisons 187
Poliomyelitis 118 et seq.
Polymyositis 200
Polyneuropathy 184
Porphyria 187
Post-concussional syndrome 99

Postencephalitic parkinsonism 120, 136
Posterior cerebral artery 124
Posterior inferior cerebellar artery 124
Post-herpetic neuralgia 148
Post-traumatic epilepsy 100
Postural control 76
Potassium utilization 202
Praxis 11, 76
Prefrontal cortex 45
Presenile dementia 135
Pressure sores 180
Progressive muscular atrophy 167
Progressive supranuclear palsy 137
Proprioception 19, 76
Pseudobulbar palsy 9, 168
Pseudohypertrophy 197
Pseudotumour cerebri 132
Ptosis 25
Punch drunk syndrome 98, 135
Pupillary reflexes 30
Pupils, Argyll Robertson 35, 116
Pyramidal fibres 3
Pyridoxine 186

Queckenstedt test 56, 157

Radiculopathy 185
Radioactive brain scanning 107
Ramus communicans 24
Rebound hypoglycaemia 84
Recruitment test 71
Referred headache 143
Referred pain 25
Reflex, abdominal 78
  bladder 28
  corneal 69
  cremasteric 78
  grasp 45
  light 34
  plantar 18, 78
  pupillary 30
  stretch 16
Respiration, assisted 119, 189, 195
Reticular formation 47
Retrobulbar neuritis 174
Rigidity 14, 18, 137
Rinne's test 70
Romberg's sign 15, 164

Sagittal sinus 131
Salaam attacks 93

Index

Schilling test 165
Scotoma 30, 174, 178
Seizures—see epilepsy
Sensory cortex 21, 46, 90
Sensory suppression 46, 76
Sensory system 15
Sensory testing 75
Septic sinus thrombosis 131
Shy-Drager syndrome 137
Sinus, cavernous 131
 lateral 131
 sagittal 131
Sleep 58
Smell, sense of 29
Snellen charts 66
Spastic paraplegia 96
Spastic paraparesis 79
Spasticity 8
Speech 60
Sphenoidal ridge meningioma 104
Spinal accessory nerve 44, 73
Spinal arteries 53
Spinal cord, anatomy 52
 compression 153, 156 et seq.
 diseases 152 et seq.
Spinocerebellar degeneration 179
Spinothalamic tract 48
Spondylosis, cervical 153, 158
Squint 36
Status epilepticus 95
Stereognosis 76
Steroids 177, 189, 195, 201
Strabismus 36
Straight leg raising test 75, 182
Streptomycin 113, 152
Stroke 123
Subacute combined degeneration of spinal cord 154, 162
Sydenham's chorea 141
Sympathetic system 23
Syncope 84, 122
Syphilis 113
Syringobulbia 170
Syringomyelia 154, 169

Tabes dorsalis 114
Tardive dyskinesia 139
Taste, sense of 70
Temporal arteritis 146
Temporal lobe 47
 epilepsy 91
Tension headache 143
Thalamic syndrome 21, 47

Thalamus 21, 47
Thiamine 134, 186
Thoracic inlet syndrome 162
Thrombophlebitis 108
Thrombosis, cerebral 123
 sinus 131
Thymus 194, 195
Thyrotoxic myopathy 201
Tinnitus 43, 151
Titubation 16, 175
Todd's paralysis 90
Tone, muscle 74
Tongue 44
Transverse myelitis 155, 177
Tremor 14, 136, 141
Treponema pallidum 113
Trigeminal nerve 37, 68
Trigeminal neuralgia 147
Trochlear nerve 33, 68
Tumour headache 142
Tumour, intracranial 101 et seq., 134
 cord 153, 156
Two point discrimination 46

Ulnar neuropathy 192
Uncinate fits 91
Unconscious patient 80, 100
Unconsciousness 58

Vagus nerve 43, 72
Vascular disease 59
Vascular headache 142
Vertebral arteries 52
Vertigo 41, 151
Vestibular nerve 40
Vestibular neuronitis 152
Vestibular system 72
Virus encephalitis 120
Virus infections 117 et seq.
Vision—see optic nerve
Vit B1, Thiamine 134, 186
Vit B6, Pyroxidine 113, 186
Vit B12, Cyanocobalamin 134, 163, 186
Von Recklinghausen's disease 105, 157

Wasserman reaction 117
Weakness 8
Weber's test 71

Werdnig-Hoffman disease 203
Wernicke's encephalopathy 133, 186
Willis, circle of 50, 124, 127

Wilson's disease 139
Wrisberg, intermediate nerve of 39, 70, 150